Congenital Deafness

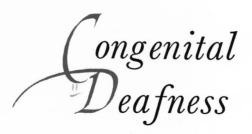

Congenital Deafness

A new approach to early detection
of deafness through a high risk register

FRANKLIN O. BLACK, M.D.
Assistant Professor of Surgery (Otolaryngology)

■

LaVONNE BERGSTROM, M.D.
Assistant Professor of Surgery (Otolaryngology)

■

MARION DOWNS, MA.
Assistant Professor of Surgery (Otolaryngology)

■

WILLIAM HEMENWAY, M.D.
Professor of Surgery
Head, Division of Otolaryngology

Colorado Associated University Press
Boulder, Colorado

Library of Congress Card Catalog Number 76-135285
ISBN 87081-005-7

From the Division of Otolaryngology, Department of Surgery
University of Colorado Medical Center
4200 East Ninth Avenue
Denver, Colorado 80220

This study partially supported by
USPH Otolaryngology Training Grant #97214
and by the
Deafness Research Foundation #67211

Contents

Acknowledgments

The authors wish to express their deep gratitude to Mrs. Page T. Jenkins for her untiring assistance in assembling reference materials for the manuscript; to Mrs. Ruth Gilbert of the Denver Veterans Administration Hospital, who procured from other libraries reference materials for the study; to Dr. John Stears, Assistant Professor of Radiology, who interpreted the petrous pyramid polytomograms and selected the x-ray illustrations used; and to the secretaries, Miss Joyce Little and Mrs. Mary Ujifusa, who typed the manuscript.

Foreword

The authors are aware that neither the validity nor the relative efficiency of a high risk register in identifying deafness at birth has been established. A great deal of study will be necessary to determine the optimum number of categories that will produce an acceptable proportion of true positives. If a high risk listing is too sensitive, it will yield an unmanageable number of false positives; if it is not inclusive enough, it will miss some hearing-handicapped infants. The ideal register would offer a compromise between the two extremes.

In the present listing we have included all the conditions which are known to have even an occasional association with deafness. It is impossible in most instances to estimate the percentage of chance that deafness will accompany the condition. The users of a register are urged to experiment with various combinations of the listing that will produce the greatest efficiency.

From our experience we are convinced that a diligent scrutiny of infants in the high risk category, plus some type of hearing screening tests, will identify most of the infants with hearing impairment at birth. It should always be remembered, however, that some hereditary hearing losses may begin after birth and progress rapidly or gradually. Therefore, vigilance should never be relaxed, and a parent's suspicion of a hearing problem should always be a sign for further investigation.

For those who wish to study the literature on high risk registers, a bibliography is given below.

References

1. Anderson, U.M., Jenss, R., Mosher, W.E., Randall, C.L., Marra, E., High risk groups—definition and identification. *New Engl. J.Med.* 273, 308-313, 1965.
2. Oppe, T.E., Risk registers for babies, *Devl. Med. Child Neurol.* 9, 13-21, 1967.
3. Richards, I.D.G. & Roberts, C.J., The "at risk" infant. *The Lancet* 2, 711-714, 1967.
4. Sheridan, M., Infants at risk for handicapping condition. *Mon. Bull. Minist. Hlth,* 21, 238-245, 1962.

Introduction

A GROWING CONCERN WITH THE NEED TO IDENTIFY hearing loss that exists at birth has focused attention on congenital ear patholo-gies. It appears that a comprehensive high risk register for deafness would be helpful to facilitate the identification of the hearing-impaired infant. Such a register should be practical enough to allow non-medical personnel such as nurses, audiologists and hospital aides to use it in the newborn nursery.

The use of a high risk register for deafness does not preclude the use of other methods of searching for the highly suspect infant. Where newborn hearing screening programs are in effect (Downs and Sterritt 1967; Downs 1969), the high risk register serves as an adjunct to screening, by encouraging more careful evaluation of those infants with a high probability of deafness. The screening personnel can also carry out the mechanics of a register, where physicians' time is limited. A register is particularly important in congenital conductive impairments because most current screening techniques may not identify more moderate losses found in congenital middle ear anomalies or milder sensori-neural losses. Infants with such losses may respond to the high levels of sound that are required for mass screening and therefore may not be identified. A high incidence of such conductive hearing losses exists in first and second arch syndromes. The register can be useful also in identifying those infants at risk for hearing losses that will develop in later life as a result of genetic factors. The ideal program would be one combining hearing screen-ing with a high risk register, because it is probable that as many as 22.5 percent

[1]

of the congenitally deaf population would not be identified by a high risk register alone.

The literature concerned with congenital deafness contains many audiological inaccuracies and inconsistencies. Many of the earlier papers describing syndromes associated with hearing loss reported "deafness" to accompany the syndrome, but did not specify the type of loss (conductive or sensori-neural), degree of loss (in decibels), or functional aspects of the loss (e.g., speech discrimination ability). Clinics with a high case load of congenital birth defects often find that a good audiological workup may reveal normal hearing in children with syndromes previously reported to be associated with deafness. Conversely, in some syndromes previously thought to be unaccompanied by hearing loss, careful audiological study will show that true hearing loss exists. Usually such syndromes involve severe multiple defects and/or mental retardation, making it difficult to evaluate the hearing. In the present high risk listing an attempt has been made to identify such discrepancies and inaccuracies, insofar as the authors' clinical experience permits.

A high risk listing is most comprehensible in terms of the relationships between genetic factors, temporal bone pathology, and clinical disease entities. These relationships are complex and can be classified in several ways: 1) genetically, 2) pathologically, and 3) by clinical findings and history.

Genetic Classification

From Proctor (1967) a classification of congenital hereditary deafness*
evolves as follows:

Hereditary deafness .... 50% of all deafness
    A. Recessive hereditary deafness 90%
    B. Dominant hereditary deafness 10%

Another way of looking at genetic, as compared with acquired deafness,
is outlined by Fraser (1964), who apportions all deafness as follows:

Apportionment of all Deafness

Hereditary
  Autosomal recessive
    With retinitis pigmentosa 3%
    With goiter 7.5%
    With abnormal ECG 1%
    Others 26%
  Autosomal dominant
    With pigmentary abnormalities 2.5%
    Without pigmentary abnormalities 10%
    Sex-linked (61% acquired later) 1.5%
                 Total genetic 51.5%

Acquired
  Prenatally 6%
  Perinatally (including prematurity) 10%
  Postnatally 30%

                  Total acquired 46%

Congenital malformation 2.5%

*For the purpose of this study we interpret congenital deafness as *hearing loss occurring
as a result of factors present before or at the time of birth.* Some genetically determined
hearing losses may not become manifest until later in life, but the genetic abnormality is
present at conception. Therefore, these losses are congenital in our frame of reference.
Although the main purpose of a high risk register is to permit early identification and habilitation, it is equally important to monitor those whose losses may occur later in life.

Many genes are involved in hereditary deafness and therefore the chance is small that both parents will carry the identical gene for deafness. However, the incidence of consanguinity is greatly increased among the normal hearing parents of deaf children. This factor tends to make manifest those recessive deafness traits carried by consanguineous parents. In addition, deaf persons tend to marry other deaf persons, but this factor may give only a slightly increased overall risk of deafness in their children, due to the small chance that two such persons would be affected by the same genetic deafness. If the *same* recessive gene is carried by *each* normal hearing parent, theoretically one-fourth of the offspring would be affected and one-half would be carriers. However, if *both* parents are *overtly* affected by the same recessive type of hereditary deafness, they are homozygous for the trait, and, therefore, all their children will be affected and capable of passing the trait on to some of their offspring in turn.

In dominant inheritance the affected person is usually heterozygous for the trait, which puts one-half of his offspring at risk of being affected. The normal offspring are not carriers. The very rare instance of a heterozygous dominant marrying a heterozygous or homozygous recessive is a situation in which two different traits of deafness are, by definition, involved. In this instance half of the children will be deaf, but from one-half to all of the children will be carriers of the recessive deafness trait. In the rare instance in which one parent with dominant deafness is homozygous, all of his children would be affected.

Sex-linked inheritance may be either recessive or dominant. All sex-linked defects are carried on the X chromosome, as the Y chromosome apparently has no function in most traits. In sex-linked recessive deafness traits all males are affected if their X chromosome carries the gene for the trait, whereas females must be homozygous to show the trait. In dominant father-daughter-transmitted traits, all daughters are affected, but in dominant traits carried by the mother half of her sons and half of her daughters are affected (Brown 1967).

The recessive hereditary deafnesses comprise up to 45 percent of all congenital hearing impairments. Fifty percent of these have no associated defects that would identify the infants as suspects (Proctor 1967). Therefore, up to 22.5 percent of all congenital hearing problems will be suspected only by reference to the family history. Anyone familiar with the vagaries of obtaining a history of recessive inheritance will recognize the low probability that recessive hearing losses will be identified other than by actual testing. This fact confirms the need to screen the entire newborn population rather than just the known high risks, even though the yield is low. The probable incidence of congenital deafness is around one in 2000 live births.

[4]

Pathological Classification

In some of the genetic classifications there is a clear relationship between temporal bone pathology and the genetic type; in other classifications the relationship is clouded. Lack of information correlating temporal bone pathology with degree and type of loss, age of onset and etiology is in large part responsible for the lacunae in our knowledge. An attempt will be made herein to relate temporal bone pathology to both function and etiology. The four classical pathological types of congenital deafness will be presented as well as other known clinical entities.

I. Classical Temporal Bone Pathology
    A. *Michel Type* (Michel 1863); Agenesis of the inner ear
        1. *Pathological findings*
        Total absence of the inner ear and auditory nerves. The authors have identified a possible Michel type in a living three-year-old congenitally deaf child. Polytomograms showed agenesis of the labyrinth (see Figure 1).
        2. *Audiological considerations*
        Audiogram should show no hearing but may reveal responses to vibratory sensation in the low frequencies at high intensity levels. No true hearing is possible; therefore, an amplification program will not be fruitful.
        3. *Etiological correlation*
        Very uncertain correlation with hereditary types. The family history was completely negative in the authors' case. Maternal ingestion of Thalidomide during pregnancy has been associated with this type of pathology. Nearly complete agenesis of the inner ear was reported in one case of Klippel-Feil deformity (McLay and Maran 1969), which is a recessive trait.
    B. *Mondini Type* (Mondini 1791; Fraser 1926-27): Bony and membranous labyrinthine dysgenesis
        1. *Pathological findings* (see Figure 2A)
          a. Malformations of bony labyrinth
          b. Cochlea may be flattened, anomalous and lack coils; usually only basal turn is present (see Figures 2B and 2C)

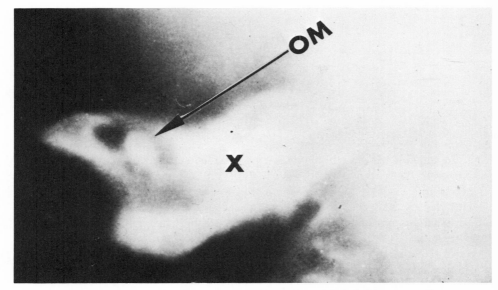

Figure 1 - Petrous pyramid polytomogram, right ear. Michel deformity of inner ear. OM is ossicular mass. Solid radio-opaque area marked with an X is that of undeveloped inner ear.
University of Colorado Medical Center

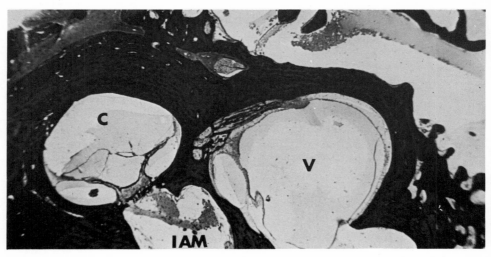

Figure 2A - Histopathologic section of inner ear showing Mondini-type deformity. C is rudimentary cochlea. The internal auditory meatus (IAM) contains normal appearing cochlear, vestibular and facial nerves. The vestibule (V) contains a large, deformed utricle.
Attributed to J.S. Fraser, 1927, by H.F. Schuknecht, *Deafness in Childhood*, Vanderbilt University Press, 1967. Used by permission.

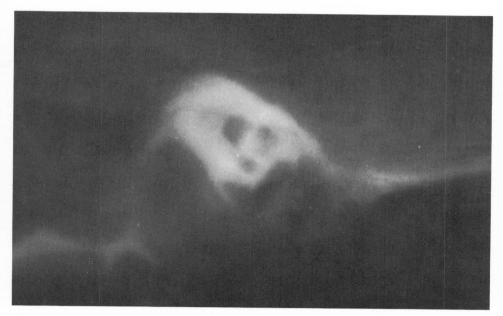

Figure 2B - Petrous pyramid polytomogram showing Mondini malformation. The flattened right cochlea with deficient coil formation is shown from the lateral aspect as compared with normal left cochlea (2C). Semicircular canals were absent. University of Colorado Medical Center

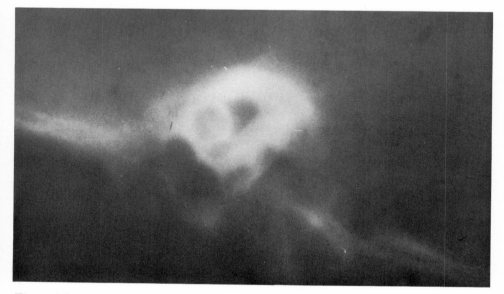

Figure 2C - Normal left cochlea.
University of Colorado Medical Center

c. Vestibular labyrinth may be deformed

d. Spiral ganglion cells variable but usually present
   Higher auditory pathways normal

2. *Audiological considerations*

   In the authors' case (Figure 3) little or no residual hearing was found, and no useful hearing function was observed.   However, multiple central nervous system dysfunctions were present, clouding the picture.   Nonetheless, true residual peripheral hearing is theoretically possible because of the likelihood of normal auditory pathways, and amplification should be utilized.   The deafness has been erroneously described as being progressive.

3. *Etiological correlation*

   There is poor correlation with hereditary types.   It has been assumed to be associated with dominant deafness.   It is sometimes associated with maternal Thalidomide ingestion (Lindeman 1967).

C. *Scheibe Type* (Scheibe 1892): Cochleo-saccular degeneration

   1. *Pathological findings* (see Figure 4)

      a. Organ of Corti degenerated, most markedly in basal coil; also saccule degeneration

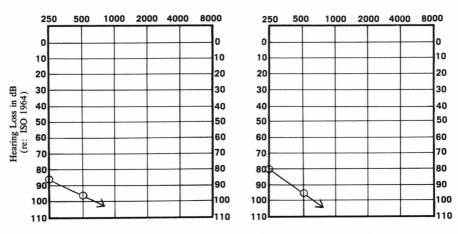

Figure 3 - Audiogram of a child with Mondini pathology.   The fragments of hearing probably represent true function.

University of Colorado Medical Center

b. Abnormalities of stria vascularis, tectorial membrane, and Reissner's membrance.
c. Normal auditory pathway beyond spiral ganglion
d. Possible vestibular effects as in retinitis pigmentosa (Siebenmann and Bing 1907). No vestibular symptoms are present in Waardenburg's syndrome which also shows Scheibe-type pathology (Waardenburg 1951; Fisch 1959).

2. *Audiological considerations*

The audiogram can be expected to show residual hearing mainly in the lower frequencies. As some hair cells may be identified histologically and the auditory pathways may be normal, the audiogram can represent true peripheral hearing which can be utilized in an amplification program.

3. *Etiological correlation*

Well-established correlation with certain recessive hereditary deafness syndromes. Exception: Waardenburg's syndrome, which resembles this type even though the syndrome is dominant (Proctor

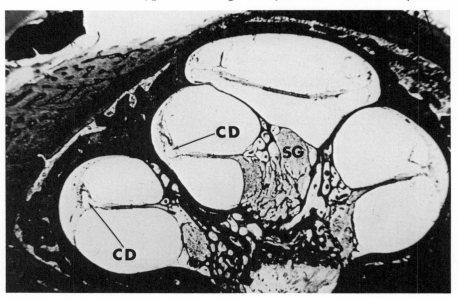

Figure 4 - Scheibe type of inner ear deformity (cochleo-saccular aplasia). Note the poorly developed cochlear duct (CD) and the normal spiral ganglion (SG). The abnormal saccule is not shown.
From Schuknecht, H.F., *Deafness in Childhood,* Vanderbilt University Press, 1967 (courtesy of Prof. L. Ruedi, Zurich, Switzerland).

[9]

1967). Also seen in deafness due to viral endolabyrinthitis, caused by measles, mumps or rubella (Hemenway and Bergstrom 1967).

D. *Alexander Type* (Alexander 1904): Membranous and cochlear dysgenesis

1. *Pathological findings*
   a. Incomplete membranous cochlear development
   b. Intact spiral ganglion and eighth nerve

2. *Audiological considerations* (see Figure 5)
   Sensori-neural hearing loss, high-tone in nature, or loss with basin-shaped audiogram (Lindsay 1967). Prospects are good for amplification and habilitation because of intact auditory pathways.

3. *Etiological correlation*
   Hereditary hearing loss, presumably dominant

Other useful pathological classifications have been reported:

Altmann (1968) observed that the pathological changes in temporal bones from cases of congenital deafness are of two basic types:

1. Regressive changes in the epithelial structures of the cochlear duct, the saccule and occasionally the utricle, their nerves, ganglia and central pathways

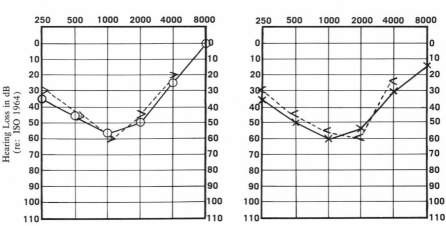

Figure 5 - Typical audiogram of dominant hereditary loss with Alexander type of pathology. Often several members of a family may have similar losses. University of Colorado Medical Center

2. Evident anatomical anomalies of the cochlea and sometimes also of the other parts of the inner ear

The first group resembles changes found in healed mild serous or viral labyrinthitis while the second group represents purely degenerative atrophic changes. Altmann hypothesizes that the changes found in both groups result from malfunction of the stria vascularis.

Schuknecht (1967) classifies hereditary sensori-neural loss into:
1. Aplasias, characterized by varying degrees of incomplete development of the inner ear
2. Heredo-degenerations, characterized by progressive loss of hearing after the inner ear has developed normally
3. Chromosomal aberrations. Subjects with chromosomal aberrations and deafness rarely live long enough for thorough audiological evaluation. Anatomically they may manifest hypoplasias (Kos et al. 1966; Sando et al. 1970; Black et al. 1970).

II. Clinical Entities Associated with Known Temporal Bone Pathologies
   A. *Infections*
      1. *Bacterial meningitis and meningoencephalitis* (This entity may be congenital as a result of sepsis associated with premature rupture of the fetal membranes) (see Figures 6A and 6B)
         a. Temporal bone pathology (Lindsay 1967; Paparella and Suguira 1967)
            (1) Cochlear neurons and organ of Corti destroyed extensively or completely by infection
            (2) Stria vascularis and tectorial membrane damaged or destroyed
            (3) Vestibular system damaged or obliterated
            (4) Inner ear and labyrinthine spaces become filled first with white cells, then serofibrinous exudates; liquefaction necrosis ensues. The spaces are then filled with fibrous tissue and varying degrees of new bone.
         b. Audiological considerations
            (1) There is no true hearing when the pathology described above is present. Where low frequency responses are seen they must represent vibratory sensation. However, the authors have seen cases following recovery from meningitis with mild to moderate sensori-neural hearing losses (see Figure 7). No temporal bone findings are known in such cases, and it is uncertain whether the losses are caused by the infection, by ototoxic drugs, or by other factors.

[11]

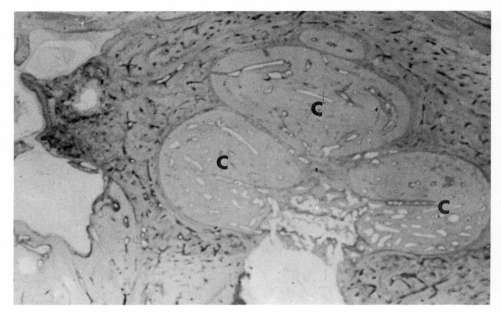

Figure 6A - Temporal bone histopathology of a patient who had had meningitis. Cochlea (C) entirely filled with new bone.
Courtesy of J.R. Lindsay, M.D., University of Chicago.

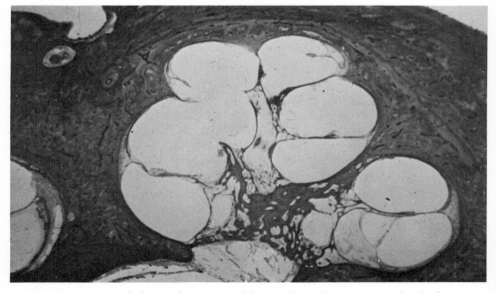

Figure 6B - Histopathology of a temporal bone of another patient who had meningitis. Note complete destruction of organ of Corti and cochlear nerve fibers.
University of Colorado Medical Center

(2) Amplification is useless when the inner ear destruction described above occurs. Where mild to severe sensori-neural losses can be demonstrated, amplification is beneficial in proportion to the amount of residual hearing.

2. *Endolymphatic labyrinthitis of viral origin* (includes maternal rubella, measles, and mumps)

    a. Temporal bone pathology (Kelemen 1966a; Hemenway and Bergstrom 1967; Lindsay 1967; Bordley et al. 1967; Alford 1968)

        (1) Organ of Corti degenerated, most markedly at basal turns; also saccule degenerated

        (2) Abnormalities of stria vascularis, tectorial membrane, Reissner's membrane, more marked at basal turn (Figure 8)

        (3) First order cochlear neurons degenerated in proportion to destruction of supporting cells of organ of Corti. Normal auditory pathways beyond spiral ganglion

        (4) Occasional involvement of entire vestibular system, especially in mumps

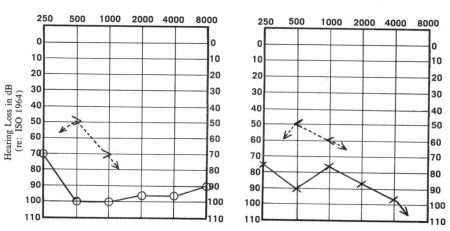

Figure 7 - Audiogram of a 10-year-old child two years after recovery from meningitis. Hearing aid was applied in left ear immediately following recovery, and discrimination improved from 0% to 44%.
University of Colorado Medical Center

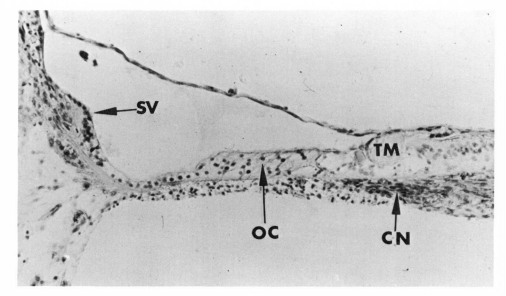

Figure 8 - Temporal bone histopathology typical of viral endolabyrinthitis (rubella).
Note atrophy of the stria vascularis (SV), degeneration of the hair cells of the organ
of Corti (OC), and the rolled up tectorial membrane (TM). Cochlear nerve fibers
(CN) are preserved.
University of Colorado Medical Center

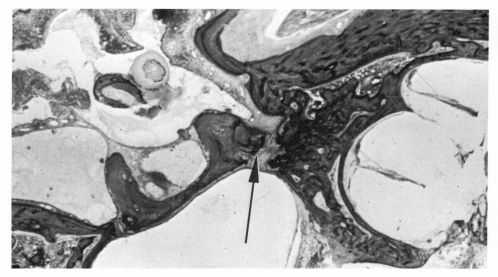

Figure 9 - Histopathology of rubella temporal bone showing fixation of the stapes
footplate (arrow).
From W.G. Hemenway et al., *Archiv. Klin. exp. Ohr. -Nas.- u- Kehlk.* 1969.

(5) One case of deafness from maternal rubella reported in the authors' clinic (Hemenway et al. 1969), in which congenital fixation of the footplate was found in addition to cochleo-saccular pathology (see Figure 9).

b. Audiological considerations

(1) Audiograms vary from mild to profound, saucer-shaped or high-tone sensori-neural losses.

(2) As neural pathways are likely to be intact, any residual hearing can be utilized in an amplification program, success depending on the degree of intactness of the nervous system.

(3) An audiogram and corresponding speech reception findings are shown in Figure 10. These are typical of many of the cases of rubella deafness seen clinically. It is thought that the bone conduction thresholds shown here represent true cochlear reserve, in view of the good functional use of hearing displayed. Such findings may correlate with the type of pathology shown in Figures 8 and 9, involving organ of Corti degeneration, stapes fixation but preservation of cochlear nerve fibers. In all cases where good hearing function resulted, amplification and training were instituted well before one year of age.

3. *Congenital syphilitic infection*

a. Temporal bone pathology (Mayer and Fraser 1936; Goodhill 1939; Perlman and Leek 1952; Karmody and Schuknecht 1966)

(1) Gummata of the otic capsule

(2) Osteomyelitis

(3) Endolymphatic hydrops

(4) Degeneration of the organ of Corti and the maculae and cristae of the vestibular end organs

(5) Bony and fibrous tissue invasion of the endolymphatic and perilymphatic spaces

(6) Loss of spiral ganglion cells, cochlear and vestibular and neural atrophy

(7) Serous labyrinthitis

(8) Deformities of the stapes footplate

(9) Periostitis

(10) Vascular changes

(11) Endolymphatic-perilymphatic fistulae

b. Audiological considerations

In Karmody and Schuknecht's series (1966), 37 percent developed hearing symptoms in early childhood. Onset of hearing

[15]

loss is usually sudden, bilaterally symmetrical, severe to profound, and not accompanied by marked vestibular manifestations (see Figure 11). Poor hearing function and limited use of hearing aid can be expected due to neural atrophy.

B. *Chromosomal Abnormalities* (Kos et al. 1966; Kelemen 1966a)

    1. *The Trisomies*

        a. Trisomy 13-15 (D)

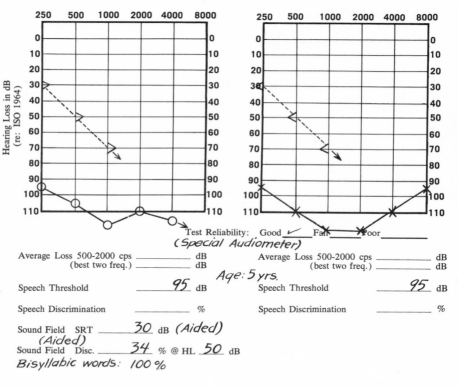

Figure 10 - Audiogram of a 5-year-old child with deafness from rubella syndrome. The bone conduction threshholds are considered to represent valid hearing. The discrimination score of 34% was obtained with adult PB list. University of Colorado Medical Center

[16]

(1) Temporal bone pathology (when sensori-neural loss is present)
  (a) Cochlea and saccule degenerated. Organ of Corti absent or replaced by fibrous tissue
  (b) Tectorial membrane, Reissner's membrane, stria vascularis degenerated
  (c) Spiral ganglion intact
  (d) Utricle and semicircular canals intact
(2) Audiological considerations
  These infants fail to thrive and most expire within a few months. Deafness without usable hearing must be expected when a sensori-neural loss is present in combination with the described pathology. First arch anomalies often accompany the syndrome: abnormal pinnae, cleft lip and/or palate, external canal atresia. One such case tested by the authors gave normal bone conduction responses but air conduction was reduced by 60–70 dB; another case gave normal responses.

b. Trisomy 18 (E)
  (1) Temporal bone pathology (Kos et al. 1966; Sando et al. 1970) (see Figures 12A and 12B)
    (a) Bony modiolus incompletely developed, spiral ganglion absent
    (b) Organ of Corti and vestibular structures normal, but

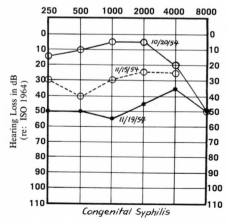

RIGHT EAR
FREQUENCY IN CYCLES PER SECOND

Congenital Syphilis

Figure 11 - Audiogram of hearing loss due to congenital syphilis, showing changes in hearing level over a short period of time.

From Karmody, C.S. and Schuknecht, H.F., *Arch. Otolaryng.* 83, 1966. Reproduced by permission.

[17]

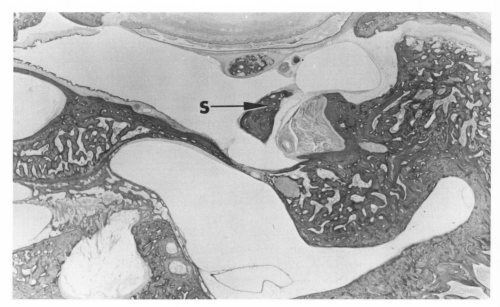

Figure 12A - Histopathology of a temporal bone of an infant who had the trisomy 18 syndrome. Note the abnormal stapes (S).
Courtesy of Dr. Isamu Sando, University of Colorado Medical Center

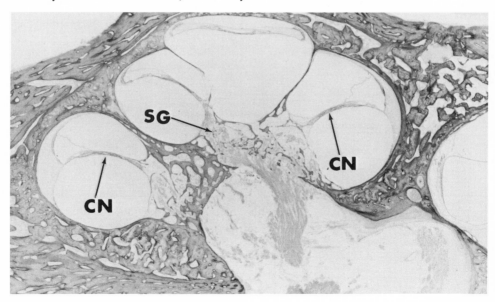

Figure 12B - Histopathology of inner ear, trisomy 18. Note fairly normal cochlear nerve (CN) and spiral ganglion cells (SG).
University of Colorado Medical Center

cochlea flattened and scala communis found between middle and apical turns

(c) Only a few ganglion cells remain at basal end of cochlea
(d) Stenosis of external auditory canal
(e) Multiple ossicular anomalies
(f) Absence of portions of the vestibular labyrinth

(2) Audiological considerations

"Infant responded to loud sounds" (Kos et al. 1966). Presumably, usable hearing can be present.

2. *Turner's syndrome* (Szpunar and Rybak 1968)

a. Pathology

No postmortem temporal bone studies are available. X-rays have revealed hypocellular mastoids. One case has been reported in which a malformation of the stapes was found at operation. Otitis media seems common in these cases.

b. Audiological considerations

Reported audiograms show mild to moderate conductive losses or basin-shaped sensori-neural loss (Szpunar and Rybak 1968; Anderson and Wedenberg 1968).

C. *Iatrogenic Toxic Deafness* (Robinson and Cambon 1964; Jorgensen and Kristensen 1964; Hawkins 1967a and b)

1. *Ototoxic drugs* (including kanamycin, neomycin, dihydrostreptomycin, streptomycin and others). Congenital deafness may result when the drugs are administered during pregnancy to the mother, e.g., streptomycin is known to cross the placental barrier and cause hearing loss in the infant (Robinson and Cambon 1964).

a. Temporal bone pathology (inferred from adult cases and animal studies)

(1) Outer hair cells damaged predominantly, but inner hair cells can also be affected. Greater damage usually in basal turns (see Figures 13A, B and C).

b. Audiological considerations

(1) Audiogram may show a flat, high-tone or saucer-shaped configuration, mild to profound sensori-neural hearing loss.

(2) Amplification is usually beneficial where sufficient residual hearing is present, despite unusually difficult initial adjustment in adults (see Figure 14). The audiogram shown is that of the 12-year-old boy whose temporal bone appears in Figure 13. Note that despite hair cell damage, the fairly intact nerve fibers suggest good potential use of the residual hearing.

[19]

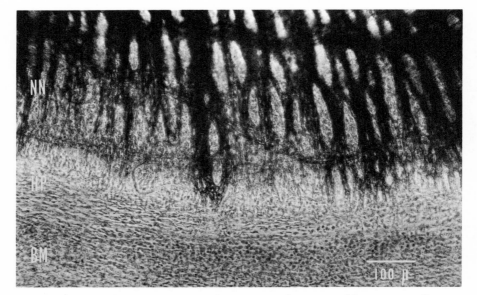

Figure 13A - Surface preparation of inner ear of 12-year-old patient with neomycin ototoxicity and renal insufficiency. Upper basal turn showing loss of Corti's organ from basilar membrane (BM) and degeneration of myelinated nerve fibers near the habenula perforata (HP).
Courtesy of Joseph E. Hawkins, Jr., Ph.D., Kresge Hearing Research Institute, University of Michigan.

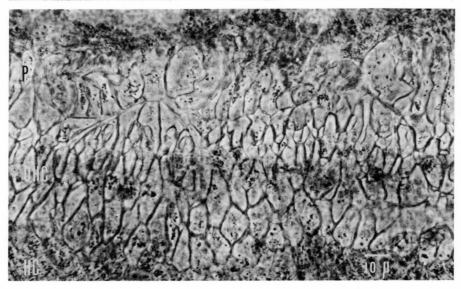

Figure 13B - Middle turn, showing severe scarring and distortion of the normal pattern of the pillars (P), characteristic of neomycin damage. Phalangeal scars replace the outer hair cells (OHC). HC—Hensen's cells.
Courtesy of Joseph E. Hawkins, Jr., Ph.D., Kresge Hearing Research Institute, University of Michigan.

2. *Fetal toxicity* (Jorgensen and Kristensen 1964)
   a. Thalidomide.   Reported as occurring from Thalidomide administered to mother during pregnancy.
      (1) Temporal bone findings
          (a) Michel or Mondini type pathology
          (b) Some middle ear anomalies
          (c) Seventh and eighth nerves absent
      (2) Audiological findings
          Approximately 75 percent can be expected to have moderate to profound sensori-neural losses, 25 percent complete conductive losses (d'Avignon and Barr 1964).
   b. Chloroquine (Matz and Naunton 1968).   Reported as causing deafness of child when given to mother during first trimester of pregnancy.
      (1) Temporal bone findings
          Organ of Corti absent in all turns and no inner or outer

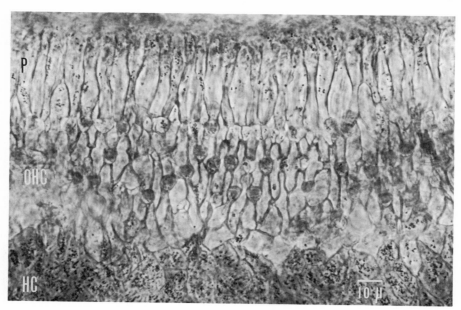

Figure 13C - Apical turn with many outer hair cells (OHC) surviving and bearing sterocilia.   All inner hair cells have disappeared.   The pillars show only moderate scarring and irregularity of pattern.   HC—Hensen's cells.
Courtesy of Joseph E. Hawkins, Jr., Ph.D., Kresge Hearing Research Institute, University of Michigan.

hair cells or supporting cells visible. Decreased number of ganglion cells but a normal auditory nerve.

    (2) Audiological considerations

        Profound bilateral sensori-neural hearing loss and no speech developed in the case reported.

D. *Congenital Anomalies* (McKenzie 1958; Hough 1958; Guilford 1967; Sando et al. 1968)

Middle ear anomalies can occur sporadically in isolated form, or with associated external ear or somatic anomalies. When associated with first and second arch syndromes, such anomalies are considered to be dominantly inherited and typically occur in Pierre Robin and Treacher Collins syndromes.

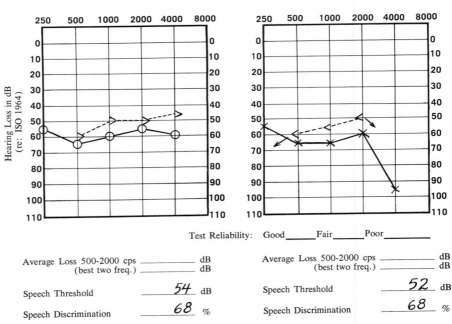

Figure 14 - Audiogram of 12-year-old child with hearing loss due to neomycin toxicity. Note the fairly adequate discrimination scores in relation to the great destruction of hair cells shown in Figures 13A & B.

University of Colorado Medical Center

1. *Temporal bone findings*
   a. Without associated anomalies
      (1) Congenital fixed footplate
      (2) Isolated ossicular anomalies
      (3) Absence of oval window (Tabor 1961; Pou 1963; Nakamura and Sando 1966)
   b. With external ear anomalies, unilateral or bilateral: atresia or stenosis of external canal, microtia, low-set pinnae (Mengel et al. 1969)
      (1) Complete or partial absence of middle ear structures. Tympanum, incus and stapes may be fused; columellar stapes and fixed footplate may occur (see Figure 15).
      (2) Inner ear abnormalities (Naunton and Valvassori 1968)
   c. With associated first or second arch syndromes: complete or partial absence of middle ear structures as in "b"
   d. With rubella: abnormal stapes reported at operation by Richards

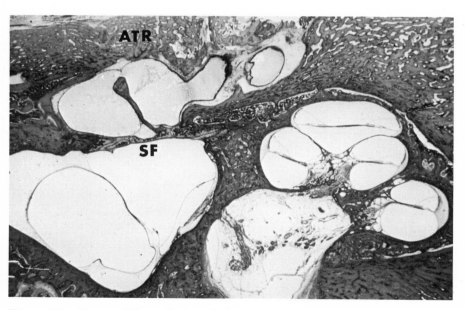

Figure 15 - Temporal bone histopathology, Treacher Collins syndrome. Note fixation of cartilaginous stapes footplate (SF) and atresia of external auditory canal (ATR).
From I. Sando et al. *Trans. Amer. Acad. Ophthal. & Otol.* 1968.

(1964) and stapedial fixation by Hemenway et al. (1969) (see Figure 9)

2. *Audiological considerations*

    a. Maximum conductive hearing loss (40-65 dB air-bone gap). Occasionally associated with sensori-neural loss.

    b. Auditory habilitation prognosis excellent. Bone conduction hearing aid can be applied shortly after birth if ear canal anomalies do not permit application of air conduction instrument. If inner ear is also anomalous there may be normal or abnormal bone conduction (Naunton and Valvassori 1968).

E. *Connective Tissue Disorders*

1. *Osteogenesis imperfecta* (Altmann 1962; Opheim 1968; Hall and Rφhrt 1968)

    a. *Temporal bone findings* (Altmann 1962)

Diminished or immature bone formation in otic capsule and ossicles. Oval window involvement and stapes fixation have been believed to be due to pathology identical to otosclerosis, but Altmann denies this. Degeneration of the stapes crura so that no contact is possible between crura and footplate, has been described (Opheim 1968; Hall and Rφhrt 1968)

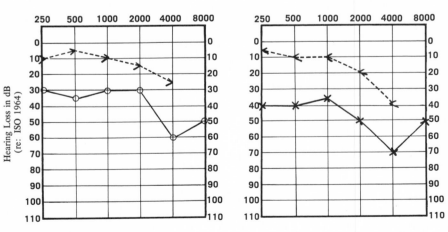

Figure 16A - Audiogram of 35-year-old man with osteogenesis imperfecta. University of Colorado Medical Center

b. *Audiological considerations*

Conductive hearing loss when middle ear pathology is present. Sensori-neural hearing loss has also been demonstrated (see Figures 16A and 16B)

2. *Hurler's syndrome (gargoylism) (Wolff 1942; Kelemen 1966b; Singleton 1968)*

a. *Temporal bone findings*

Persistent mesenchyme in the middle ear, signs of chronic otitis media, ossicular joint fusion, dense mastoids, mucopolysaccharide deposits, gargoyle cells, collapsed cochlear duct.

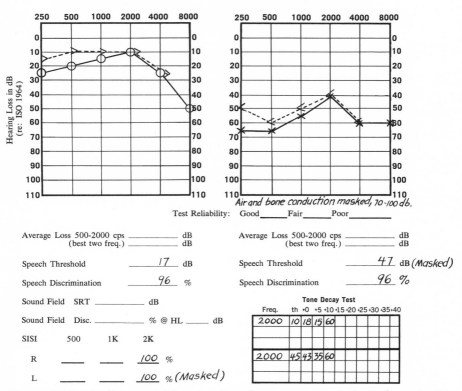

Figure 16B - Audiogram of hearing loss from osteogenesis imperfecta in 30-year-old woman. Patient had not been aware of any loss prior to this time. University of Colorado Medical Center

b. *Audiological considerations*

Mild, probably conductive loss of 20-40 dB found in children too severely retarded to evaluate more satisfactorily and mild high-tone sensori-neural loss in others (Singleton 1968). A case of the authors' is shown in Figure 17.

3. *Achondroplasia*

a. *Temporal bone findings*: Absence of cartilage in enchondral bone layer, deformed bony labyrinth (Schuknecht 1967)

b. *Audiological findings*: Conductive hearing loss of 40-70 dB due to serous otitis media (Yarington and Sprinkle 1967)

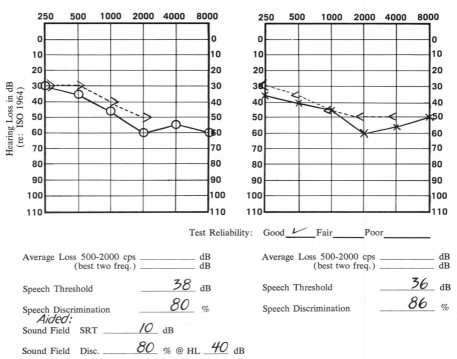

Figure 17 - Audiogram of 8-year-old child with Hunter-Hurler's syndrome. Hearing aids are worn with good results.
University of Colorado Medical Center

[26]

F. *Cardio-auditory Syndrome of Jervell and Lange-Nielsen* (Friedman et al. 1965)
   1. *Temporal bone findings*
      a. Similar to Scheibe malformation
      b. Periodic-acid-Schiff-positive deposits in the membranous labyrinth
   2. *Audiological considerations*
      Profound sensori-neural hearing loss (Jervell and Lange-Nielsen 1957). One two-day-old infant tested by authors shortly before it expired unexpectedly showed no response to any stimuli.
G. *Skeletal Defects*
   1. *Klippel-Feil syndrome* (McLay and Maran 1969)
      a. Temporal bone findings: Narrowed middle ear space, deformed ossicles, narrow oval window niche, rudimentary egg-shaped cyst representing the cochlea. The eighth nerve was absent.
      b. Audiological findings: Conductive and profound sensori-neural losses have been reported (McLay and Maran 1969) (see Figure 18).
   2. *Treacher Collins syndrome* (Sando et al. 1968)
      a. Temporal bone findings: Atresia of the external auditory canal,

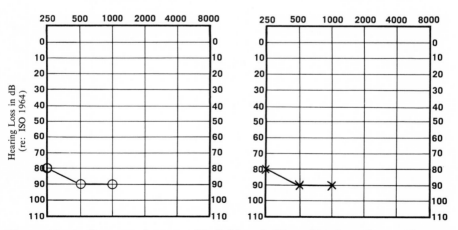

Figure 18 - Audiogram of 6-year-old child with Klippel-Feil syndrome. Hearing aid was applied at early age with successful use.
University of Colorado Medical Center

[27]

poorly developed middle ear, absent malleus and incus, abnormal stapes, absent tensor tympani and stapedius muscles, aberrant course of the facial nerve, hair cell loss in the basal turn of the cochlea, large cochlear aqueduct, abnormalities of the bony and membranous vestibular labyrinth (see Figure 15)

   b. Audiological considerations: Complete conductive loss (see Figure 19)

III. Clinical Entities Whose Pathology is Still in Doubt
   A. *Erythroblastosis Fetalis* (Goodhill 1967; Carhart 1967)
      1. *Temporal bone pathology*: No pathological reports are known in which good audiological studies were available. The pathology was originally thought to occur in the cochlear nucleus, but more recent reports point to cochlear pathology.

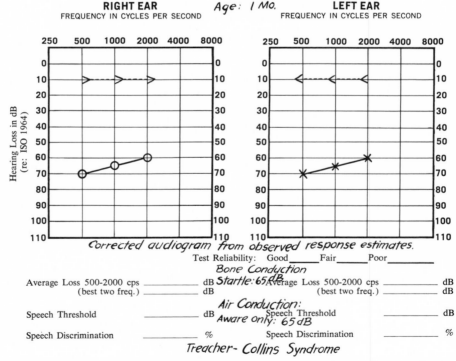

Figure 19 - Audiogram of 1-month-old child with Treacher Collins syndrome. Threshholds were estimated by correcting response levels with normative index for age.

University of Colorado Medical Center

[28]

2. *Audiological considerations*

a. Mild to profound sensori-neural hearing losses, most typically a moderately severe S-shaped curve

b. Where no severe central nervous system dysfunction exists, amplification is usually greatly beneficial (see Figure 20).

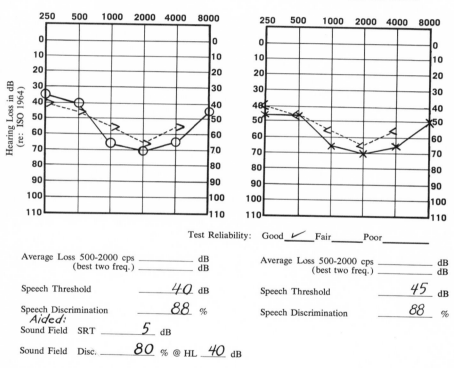

UNIVERSITY OF COLORADO MEDICAL CENTER
COLORADO GENERAL HOSPITAL

Figure 20 - Audiogram of 17-year-old female with hearing loss from maternal Rh incompatibility. Hearing aid was applied at age 2, and this girl attended regular school classes throughout her school years, achieving A average in accelerated groups.

University of Colorado Medical Center

Classification by Clinical Findings and History

The classification which appears to us to be most useful in the actual search for congenital deafness is one based on a combination of clinical findings and history. It is this kind of classification that forms the basis of the high risk listing which follows. The listing by observable symptoms may allow even the non-professional person to recognize defects concomitant with deafness and to allow such a person to identify an infant for suspicion.

The clinical categories of conditions which may be accompanied by hearing loss are:

    I. Overt (genetic)
       Easily visualized abnormalities
    II. Occult (genetic)
       Abnormalities that can be identified or suggested only by:
       1. Special physical examination
       2. Family history
    III. Congenital acquired deafness of prenatal, perinatal or neonatal origin

  I. Overt Defects Associated With Deafness
    Not all of the associated defects will be present in all cases, nor will deafness be present in all cases. For more precise descriptions, please consult references.
    A. *Skeletal and Cranial Defects*
       Infants with one or more of the following are suspect: Skull abnormalities, short neck, absent clavicles, dwarfism, malformations of extremities and digits, cleft palate (overt or submucous), underdeveloped maxillae or mandible, facial asymmetry (including facial paralysis), external ear abnormalities, low hairline, fragile bones associated with blue sclerae, knuckle pads and white nails.
       1. *Recessive hereditary syndromes*
         a. Osteogenesis imperfecta: Brittle bones (may have bony deformities from old fractures), blue sclerae of eyes (McKusick 1966). Can have either sensori-neural or conductive loss, the latter due to otosclerotic-like fixation of footplate (Alberti and Parkannen 1963) or stapes anomalies (Opheim 1968; Hall and Røhrt 1968) (see Figure 21).

[31]

b. Hurler's syndrome (gargoylism): Onset of progressive skeletal deformities after the first year of life. Mental retardation, cloudy corneas, blindness, thick eyebrows, stuffy nose, puffy skin, thick coarse hair, hirsutism, big tongue, blank stare. The hearing loss may be sensori-neural or conductive, the latter due to refractory mucoid otitis media (Hurler 1919; Waardenburg 1951; Nelson 1964; Kelemen 1966; Yarington and Sprinkle 1967; Schuknecht 1967). A sex-linked form, Hunter's syndrome, is identical clinically. (Hunter 1917; Gerich 1969) (see Figure 22).

c. Morquio's disease: Dwarfism, other skeletal deformities, normal-sized head, long extremities, short trunk (Nelson 1964; Gates 1946).

d. Oto-palato-digital syndrome: Frontal bossing, prominent occiput, ocular hypertelorism (increased space between eyes), anti-mongoloid slant of eyes, fish mouth, pseudo-winged knobby scapulae, broad distal phalanges of hands and feet, cleft palate. Conductive hearing loss due to ossicular maldevelopment and serous otitis media (Buran and Duvall 1967).

e. Albers-Schonberg's syndrome (osteopetrosis): Brittle bones, intermittent facial palsy, optic atrophy, hydrocephalus, ocular nystagmus, exophthalmos. Progressive sensori-neural loss or conductive loss (Klintworth 1963; Nelson 1964).

f. Klippel-Feil syndrome: Fused cervical vertebrae, giving appearance of very short, webbed neck or of head sitting on shoulders, low posterior hairline; spina bifida and external auditory canal atresia may be present (see Figure 23). May have severe sensori-neural loss (McLay and Maran 1969) or mixed hearing loss. In the latter case slightly abnormal ossicles and an absent oval window were found at operation (Livingstone and Delahunty 1968). An unexplained conductive hearing loss with normal external and middle ear structures was described by Singh et al. (1969). See Figure 18 for authors' case with sensori-neural hearing loss (Bardadin and Siedlanowska 1955; Fickentscher 1954).

g. Cervico-oculo-acoustic syndrome: Combination of Klippel-Feil and Duane's syndrome described by Wildervanck in 1952 (Livingstone and Delahunty 1968) with the above findings of fused neck vertebrae, spina bifida occulta, abducens palsy of eye and sensori-neural deafness. X-ray studies have suggested underdevelopment of the cochlear and vestibular apparatus.

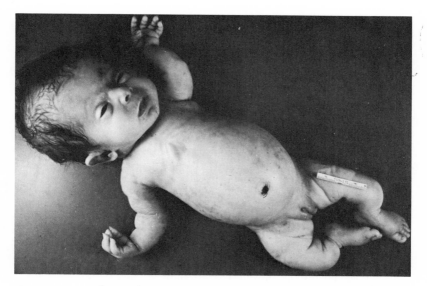

Figure 21 - Infant who died in neonatal period of osteogenesis imperfecta, congenita type.
University of Colorado Medical Center

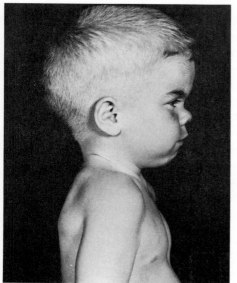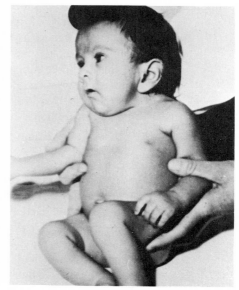

Figure 22 (*left*) - Patient showing stigmata of Hunter form of mucopolysacchari-
dosis (gargoylism). Note hirsutism, heavy eyebrows, depressed nasal bridge, thick
lips and protruding abdomen.
University of Colorado Medical Center

Figure 23 (*right*) - Infant with Klippel-Feil syndrome. Note short neck giving im-
pression that head is set directly on shoulders.
University of Colorado Medical Center

Calorics may show no reaction. Audiogram shows only a remnant of hearing up to 1500 to 3000 Hz at 90 dB (Wildervanck 1952 and 1966).

2. *Dominant hereditary syndromes*

   a. Crouzon's disease: Synostosis of cranial sutures, shallow orbits with secondary proptosis (frog-eyes), hypoplasia of maxillae with relative mandibular prognathism, parrot nose, atresia of auditory canal. Loss usually conductive but may be sensori-neural (Crouzon 1912; Clerc and Deumier 1958; Nath et al. 1964) (see Figures 24A and 24B).

   b. Cleido-cranial dysostosis: Fontanelles fail to close, facial bones underdeveloped, high arched palate, absence of clavicles, sensori-neural loss (Gorlin and Pindborg 1964) (see Figure 25).

   c. Treacher Collins syndrome: Malformation of malar and other facial bones, anti-mongoloid slant of eyes with notching of lids (colobomata), high palate, atresia and external ear malformations, middle ear anomalies. Loss usually conductive, but may be sensori-neural (Hall-Jones 1963; Maran 1964; Fernandez and Ronis 1964; Sando et al. 1968) (see Figure 26).

   d. Pierre Robin syndrome: Typical first arch syndrome. Underdevelopment and asymmetry of facial structures, cleft palate, small mandible; may have atresia of ear canal, microtia of auricles, middle ear anomalies, digital abnormalities and preauricular sweating during crying (McKenzie 1958). Complete conductive loss is present, in our experience, but others report possibility of sensori-neural loss (Sacrez et al. 1967).

   e. Apert's syndrome: Acrocephaly (tower skull), fused digits (lobster-claw hands), shallow orbits, underdeveloped maxillae, fixation of stapes causing conductive loss (Gorlin and Pindborg 1964) (see Figure 27).

   f. Achondroplasia: Dwarfism with normal-sized trunk, large head and shortened extremities, saddle nose, mandible and frontal bone protrusions. Normal intelligence. Conductive loss due to serous otitis media and/or sensori-neural deafness (Nelson 1964; Yarington and Sprinkle 1967).

   g. Knuckle pads, leukonychia and deafness: Knuckle pads, white fingernails and toenails. In one ear explored, ossicular abnormalities and dehiscent facial nerve were found. Mixed hearing loss reported (Bart and Pumphrey 1967) (see Figure 28).

   h. Myositis ossificans: Formation of true osseous tissue in skeletal

[34]

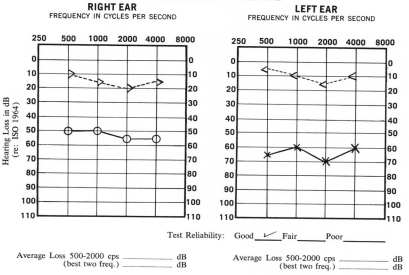

RIGHT EAR
FREQUENCY IN CYCLES PER SECOND

LEFT EAR
FREQUENCY IN CYCLES PER SECOND

Test Reliability: Good ___✓___ Fair _____ Poor _____

Average Loss 500-2000 cps _____ dB
(best two freq.) _____ dB

Average Loss 500-2000 cps _____ dB
(best two freq.) _____ dB

Speech Threshold _____ **55** dB

Speech Threshold _____ **65** dB

Figure 24A - Audiogram of 2-year-old child with Crouzon's disease. Bone conduction hearing aid was applied successfully.
University of Colorado Medical Center

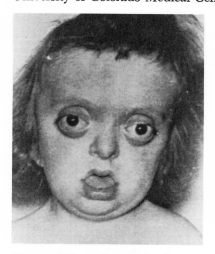

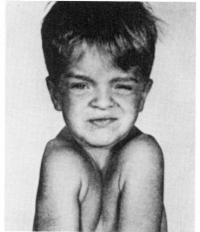

Figure 24B - Crouzon's disease. Note proptosis and bulging forehead.
From Baldwin, J., *Laryngoscope* 1968.

Figure 25 - Cleidocranial dysostosis. Note absence of clavicles and right facial weakness.
From Jaffee, S., *Laryngoscope* 1968.

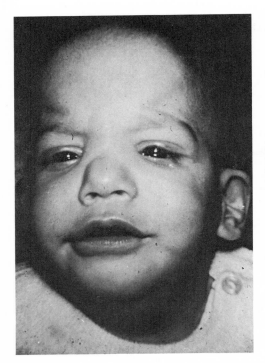

Figure 26 - Infant with Treacher Collins syndrome. Note low-set ears and anti-mongoloid obliquity of eyes. University of Colorado Medical Center

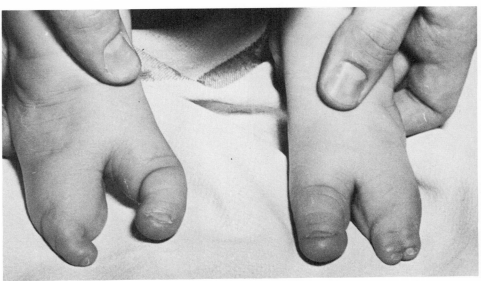

Figure 27 - Syndactyly (lobster claw hands), typical of Apert's syndrome. From Nelson, W.E., *Pediatrics*, ed. 9. W.B. Saunders Co. (courtesy of Dr. Josef Warkany)

muscle, microdactyly of great toes (70 percent) and shortened thumbs (30 percent). Both conductive and "perceptive" deafness reported (Ludman et al. 1968).

i. Symphalangism: Fusion of proximal and middle phalanges of fingers and toes giving characteristic "stiff finger and toe" appearance, prominence on medial and lateral sides of foot at the level of navicular and fifth metatarsal bones. Onset of conductive hearing loss in the first years of life. Operative exploration of the ear shows bony fusion of stapes to the petrous bone (Cushing 1916; Strasburger et al. 1965).

j. Branchial anomalies and hearing impairment: Cervical fistulas, malformed external ears, pre-auricular pits, pre-auricular appendages and mild to maximum conductive hearing loss, although sensori-neural loss has been found also. At operation the lenticular process of the incus did not reach the head of the stapes (Fourman 1955; McLaurin et al. 1966).

k. Marfan's disease: Tall, thin patient with skeletal and ocular defects. Long spidery fingers, scoliosis, hammer toe, pigeon breast, dolichocephaly, low hair line (McKusick 1966). Sensorineural or conductive deafness or both (Schilling 1936; Everberg 1959; Kelemen 1965a).

B. *Associated Eye Abnormalities*

Infants with one or more of the following are suspect: Blindness, chorioretinitis, retinal and corneal abnormalities, optic atrophy, small sunken eyes, cataracts, colobomata (clefts) of eyelids or of iris, and ocular palsy or paralysis.

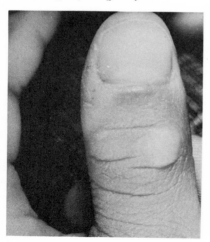

Figure 28 - Knuckle pads and white nails of knuckle pads, leukonychia and deafness syndrome.
From Bart, R.S. and Pumphrey, R.E., *N. Eng. J. Med.* 1967.

[37]

1. *Recessive hereditary syndromes*
    a. Usher's syndrome: Retinitis pigmentosa, vestibulo-cerebellar ataxia, mental retardation, chronic progressive sensori-neural deafness in 20-25 percent of all cases. Alexander type of pathology, worse at the basal turn, and spiral ganglion cell degeneration have been found (Von Graefe 1858; Usher 1914; Bochenek et al. 1958; Richards and Rundle 1959; Paparella 1969).
    b. Cockayne's syndrome: Retinal atrophy, motor disturbances, mental retardation and dwarfism. Progressive severe sensori-neural loss (Paddison et al. 1963; Remky et al. 1964–65).
    c. Alstrom's syndrome: Obesity, diabetes mellitus, retinal degeneration with loss of central vision, progressive sensori-neural deafness (Alstrom et al. 1959).
    d. Hallgren's syndrome: Retinitis pigmentosa, vestibulo-cerebellar ataxia, nystagmus, mental retardation in 24 percent. Severe congenital sensori-neural hearing loss (Hallgren 1959).
    e. Laurence-Moon-Biedl-Bardet syndrome: Retinitis pigmentosa, polydactyly, hypogenitalism, obesity, mental retardation, "deafness" in 3 percent which can also occur in otherwise normal siblings (Burn 1950).
    f. Refsum's syndrome ("Heredopathia atactica polyneuritiformis"): Retinitis pigmentosa, cerebellar ataxia, polyneuritis, electrocardiographic abnormalities, ichthyosis-type skin problem. Sensori-neural deafness (Refsum 1946, 1954; Drachman 1968). Temporal bone findings: Degeneration of Corti's organ and stria vascularis with preservation of neural structures; vestibular system (pars superior) normal (Hallpike 1967).
    g. Amalric's syndrome: Bilateral macular dystrophy; 7 percent are "deaf" (Paddison et al. 1963).
    h. Norrie's disease: Bilateral congenital blindness due to pseudo-tumor of the retina. Mental retardation, sensori-neural deafness (later, in 20-30 percent of the patients) (Warburg 1963).
    i. Leber's disease: Juvenile incomplete optic atrophy, involving mostly males. Epilepsy, ataxia, mental retardation. Clubfeet not unusual. "Deafness" reported (Francois 1961).
    j. Fehr's corneal dystrophy: Diffuse changes in cornea, blindness by 40 years, progressive sensori-neural deafness (Moro and Amidei 1957; Francois 1961).
    k. Schilder's disease: Optic atrophy, progressive spasticity, cortical blindness and "deafness", seizures, dementia, death. (Onset,

about age 5 months; course, a few weeks; if onset is later in childhood, the course is a few years) (Globus and Strauss 1928; Lichtenstein and Rosenbluth 1956).

l. Duane's syndrome: Ocular palsy (congenital fibrous replacement of rectus muscle), "deafness," auricular malformations, meatal atresia, cervical rib, torticollis, cervical spina bifida. Female, 3; Male, 2. Thalidomide implicated in some cases. Hearing loss said to be conductive. Fixed ossicular masses found at tympanotomy (Livingstone and Delahunty 1968).

m. Moebius' syndrome: Facial diplegia, lateral and/or medial rectus palsy bilaterally, "deafness" (15 percent), auricular malformation, micrognathia, absence of hands, feet, fingers or toes, mental deficiency, paralysis of tongue. Pathology: hypoplasia of brain stem nuclei. Inner ear abnormalities by x-ray in one case. Also absence of stapes, oval and round windows in one case (Livingstone and Delahunty 1968).

n. Cryptophthalmos: Eyes hidden under completely adhered eyelids, external ear malformations and conductive hearing loss (Fraser 1964).

2. *Dominant hereditary syndromes*: None known.

3. *Syndromes of doubtful hereditary origin*

a. Cogan's syndrome: It is not certain whether Cogan's syndrome is hereditary or not, and if hereditary, its mode of inheritance is unknown (Danish et al. 1963). Clinically it is characterized by vertigo, nystagmus, ataxia, keratitis and progressive sensorineural hearing loss beginning in childhood or adult life (Cogan 1945; Cody and Williams 1960). Temporal bone pathology shows degeneration of the organ of Corti, cochlear hydrops, cysts in the stria vascularis, atrophy of the spiral ganglion, deposition of connective tissue and bone in the perilymphatic spaces of the cochlea, and saccular rupture (Wolff et al. 1965).

C. *Associated Pigmentary Abnormalities*

Infants with one or more of the following are suspect: Unusually light skin, lack of pigment in iris, sclera and fundus, abnormal canthi, white forelock, different colored irises (heterochromia irides), wide root of nose, wide separation of eyes and clumps of pigment in retina.

1. *Recessive hereditary syndromes*

Albinism-deafness syndrome: Fair skin and hair, absence of pigment in iris, sclera and fundus, sensori-neural hearing loss (Ziprkowski and Adam 1964).

[39]

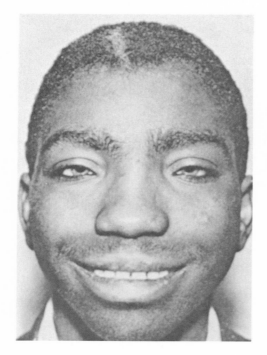

Figure 29A - Waardenburg's syndrome. Note white streak in center of hair, broad nasal root and light-colored irises in this Negro patient.

From DiGeorge, A., Olmsted, R.W. and Harley, R.D., Waardenburg's syndrome. *J. Pediat.* 57:649-669, 1960.

RIGHT EAR
FREQUENCY IN CYCLES PER SECOND
A

LEFT EAR
FREQUENCY IN CYCLES PER SECOND
B

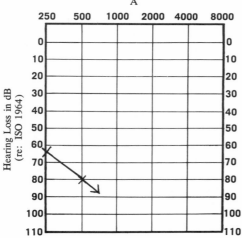
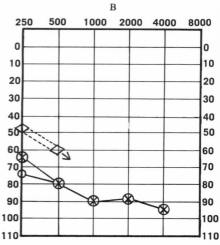

Figure 29B - Audiogram of mother (A) and daughter (B) with Waardenburg's syndrome.

Courtesy of R.E. Marcus, *Acta Otolaryng. Suppl.* 229, 1969.

2. Dominant hereditary syndromes

a. Waardenburg's syndrome: Heterochromia irides, broad nasal root, thick eyebrows, lateral displacement of medial canthi, white forelock, dappling of skin, congenital sensori-neural deafness (may be unilateral, may be progressive). Hearing loss can affect mainly low and middle frequencies, but profound deafness can also be present (Waardenburg 1951; Fisch 1959; DiGeorge et al. 1960; McKusick 1960; Proctor 1967 (see Figures 29A and 29B).

b. Albinism-deafness: Fair skin, fine hair, but eyes not affected (blue irides); can have profound sensori-neural deafness (Tietz 1963).

3. Sex-linked syndromes

a. Deafness and total albinism: severe sensori-neural deafness (Margolis 1962).

b. Deafness and partial albinism or piebaldness: areas of skin depigmentation, light blue irides, clumps of pigment throughout the retina, good vision and subtotal sensori-neural deafness (Ziprkowski and Adam 1964; Wolff, C. M. et al. 1965) (see Figure 30).

D. Associated Ectodermal Abnormalities

Infants with one or more of the following are suspect: Any unusual condition of the hair, nails, teeth, or skin; abnormal lack of sweating, oddly-shaped nose.

1. Recessive hereditary syndromes

a. Nail dystrophy and nerve deafness: Defects of hair, teeth, sebaceous glands, nails. Sensori-neural deafness (Feinmesser and Zelig 1961).

b. Pili torti and sensori-neural hearing loss: The patient has twisted hair that tends to break off easily, giving an absence of hair growth. Usually this is not recognized until the second year of life. Hypoplasia of tooth enamel is seen in some cases. The characteristic hair abnormality can be recognized by microscopic examination. The hearing loss severity tends to be positively correlated with the severity of the hair abnormality (Robinson and Johnston 1967) (see Figure 31).

2. Dominant hereditary syndromes

a. Ectodermal dysplasia, major anhidrotic type: Saddle nose, abnormal, sparse or absent teeth, no perspiration, prominent frontal bossing, sparse or brittle hair, dysphonia, congenital ozena. Moderate "deafness," present at birth or progressive in adult-

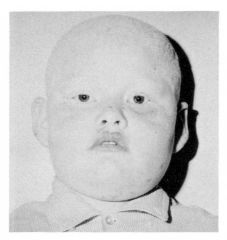

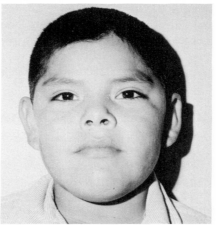

Figure 30 - Deafness and piebaldness (normal sibling in center).
From Wolff, Dolowitz and Aldous, *Arch. Otolaryng.* 1965.

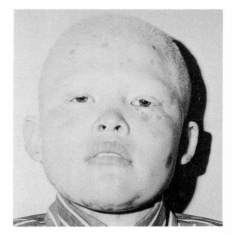

hood. Largely restricted to males (Helweg-Larsen and Ludvigsen 1946; Marshall 1958).

    b. Ectodermal dysplasia, hidrotic type: Sensori-neural deafness, polydactyly and syndactylism, small, dystrophic nails, partial loss of teeth, normal or elevated sweat electrolytes (Robinson et al. 1962).

    c. Localized von Recklinghausen's disease (neurofibromatosis), an ectodermal dysplasia: Café-au-lait spots on skin; pedunculated neurofibromas. Loss of vestibular function and sensori-neural deafness occurring later in life (Gardner and Turner 1940).

E. *Metabolic Disorders and Deafness*

  1. *Recessive hereditary disorders*

    a. Cretinism: These infants are sluggish, edematous, (especially around the eyes), have cool dry skin, large tongues, tend to have hernias, are constipated (see Figure 32). Hearing loss is perceptive or mixed (Howarth and Lloyd 1956; DeVos 1963). Temporal bone pathology shows hyperostosis of the bone of the promontory, large cochlear aqueducts and fibrous tissue obliterating the round window niche (Paparella 1969).

  2. *Dominant hereditary disorders*

  Hyperuricemia and neurologic deficits syndrome: Onset of progressive ataxia, muscle weakness and sensori-neural hearing loss in adolescence. Elevated serum uric acid precedes other manifestations, appearing at about puberty. Progressive renal disease and occasionally gout occur later. A composite audiogram of three family members with varying degrees of hearing loss is shown in Figure 33. Special hearing tests indicate a cochlear disorder (Rosenberg et al. 1970).

F. *Miscellaneous Somatic Disorders*

  1. *Trisomy 13-15 (D),* Patau's syndrome: May have low-set ears, abnormal pinnae, cleft lip and/or palate, microphthalmia, iris colo-

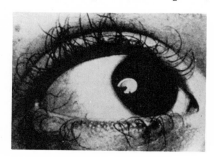

Figure 31 - Pili torti. Note long, curly eyelashes.
From Sorsby, A., *Clinical Genetics,* p. 220. Butterworth & Co. Ltd., London, 1953.

boma, mental retardation, cataracts, facial capillary hemangioma, polydactyly, sloping forehead, posterior prominence of heels, low birth weight and failure to thrive (Patau et al. 1960, Laurence 1964). Cochlear pathology and sensori-neural loss reported (Kos et al. 1966). The authors have seen one case with conductive loss and normal bone conduction.

2. *Trisomy 18 (E)*: Low-set ears, abnormal pinnae, micrognathia, high palate, mental retardation, hypertonicity, prominent occiput, flexion of index finger over third finger, equinovarus and/or rocker-bottom feet, hernias, low birth weight and failure to thrive (Miller et al. 1963; Arthur 1965; Kos et al. 1966; Warkany et al. 1966) (see Figures 34A and 34B).

3. *Rubella syndrome*: Overt manifestations may include microcephaly, congenital cataracts, purpura, and retardation. Sensori-neural deafness, possible conductive element (see Figure 10). Deafness, cardiac and cerebral lesions, bone and muscle abnormalities are occult.

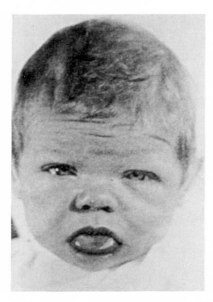

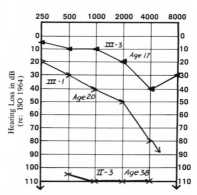

Figure 32 - Cretinism. Note large tongue, dull face and periorbital edema.

From Nelson, W.E., *Pediatrics*, ed. 6. W.B. Saunders Co.

Figure 33 - Audiograms from three family members with hyperuricemia, ataxia and deafness. Note the progression in sensori-neural loss from III-3 who is 17 years old to II-3 who is 38. University of Colorado Medical Center

[44]

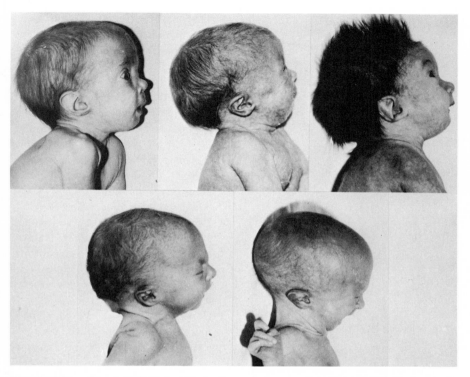

Figure 34A - Typical facial and skull appearance of patients with trisomy 18 syndrome. Note the low-set ears.
From Smith, D.W., Patau, K., Therman, E. and Inhorn, S.L., The No. 18 trisomy syndrome, *J. Pediat*. 60:513-527, 1962.

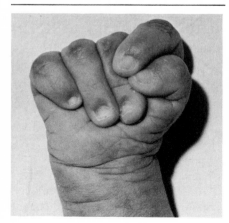

Figure 34B - Typical hand position of patients with trisomy 18 syndrome. From Smith, D.W. et al.

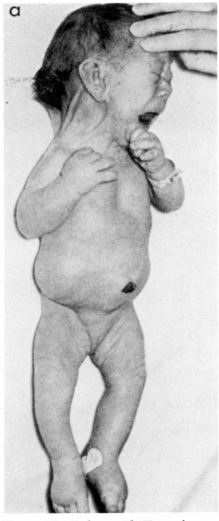

Figure 35 - Infant with Turner's syndrome. Note the webbing of the neck, the large ears and swollen dorsal aspects of the feet.
From Uchida, I.A. and Soltan, H.C., Evaluation of dermatoglyphics in medical genetics, *Ped. Clin. N. Amer.* 10:409-422, May 1963, Figure 44.

4. *Turner's syndrome*: In the newborn period these infants may show puffy hands and feet, low hairline, webbing of the neck, a shield-like chest with widely spaced nipples, numerous pigmented spots on the skin (nevi), webbing of the digits, hypoplastic nails, shortened fourth finger (see Figure 35). Hearing loss may be conductive or sensorineural (Reisman and Matheny 1969; Szpunar and Rybak 1968; Anderson and Wedenberg 1968).

5. *Trisomy 21* (Down's syndrome): Mental retardation, short stature, slanted, wide-set eyes, epicanthus, brachycephaly, short nose, and broad, flat hand are some of the characteristics.

6. *Cornelia de Lange syndrome*: These infants are small at birth, very retarded both in growth and development; hirsutism, low-pitched cry, microcephaly, eyebrows that meet in the center, small nose, low-set ears, high-arched palate, small mandible, simian palmar crease, proximally-inserted thumbs and small hands and feet are typical. Hearing loss probably is not a constant feature. Authors' cases: one with normal hearing on evoked response audiometric testing; another with conductive loss, cause as yet uncertain.

7. *Hypogammaglobulinemia*: Acquired or hereditary (recessive). Susceptibility to infection, may have acute osteomyelitis, recurrent pneumonia, refractory otitis media, multiple anomalies. Audiometry

shows conductive loss (Wallenborn 1961).

8. *Cystic fibrosis*: Pulmonary disease. Can be dominantly or recessively inherited. Intestinal atresia, peptic ulcer, and otitis media may occur. Conductive loss of varying degree (Mendelsohn and Cohen 1964).

9. *Heerfordt's disease*: Lesion of internal auditory canal and geniculate ganglion. Uveitis, parotitis, dermatitis. Moderate sensori-neural loss (Ebihara 1959).

II Occult Symptoms Associated With Deafness

Identifiable only by special physical or laboratory examination or by reference to history

A. *Congenital Renal Disorders Associated with Deafness*

1. *Recessive hereditary disorders*: None reported.

2. *Dominant hereditary syndromes*

a. Hereditary chronic nephritis

(1) Alport's syndrome: Episodic hematuria beginning in childhood, about age 10, but urinary abnormalities may be detected in infancy (microscopic hematuria and albuminuria), progressive uremia leading to renal failure, and progressive sensori-neural hearing loss; both the renal disease and the hearing loss are much more severe in males, who may die in the third decade of life. Ocular defects may be present. Two types of audiograms have been reported: descending type of curve and dip at 4000 Hz (Alport 1927; Hamburger et al. 1956; Goldbloom et al. 1957; Goldman and Haberfelde 1959; Cohen et al. 1961; Perkoff 1967) (see Figure 36).

(2) Familial hyperprolinemia

(a) Type I is characterized by hyperprolinemia, prolinuria, hydroxyprolinuria, glycinuria, renal anomalies, superimposed pyelonephritis, hematuria. Seizures, mental retardation and sensori-neural hearing loss are present in some persons with this abnormality. Audiological findings: "marked hearing loss" sensori-neural type (Schafer et al. 1962).

(b) A second type shows ichthyosis in addition to above findings. Sensori-neural hearing losses ranging from mild, high-frequency losses to moderate or profound losses can be found (Goyer et al. 1968).

(3) Urticaria, deafness and amyloidosis (Muckle and Wells

[47]

1962): Onset in adolescence of recurrent bouts of chills, fever, malaise, urticaria and progressive sensori-neural hearing loss. Later onset of progressive nephropathy due to amyloidosis. Temporal bone findings: absence of organ of Corti and vestibular sensory epithelium, atrophy of the cochlear nerve, ossification of the basilar membrane (see Figure 37) (Andersen et al. 1967).

(4) Congenital renal and ear anomalies

    (a) Microtia or anotia, under-developed facial bones and renal anomalies on the same side of the body (Taylor 1965).

    (b) Nephrosis, deafness, urinary tract and middle ear malformations, shortening and broadening of the distal portions of the thumbs and great toes, bifid uvula (Braun and Bayer 1962).

(5) Chronic renal disease and ototoxic drug administration (Beaney 1964). Some patients with diminished renal function have been given ototoxic drugs. The drug is excreted more slowly by the diseased kidneys and blood levels of the drug may remain high for a prolonged time. It is believed that the hair cells of the inner ear may, therefore, be exposed

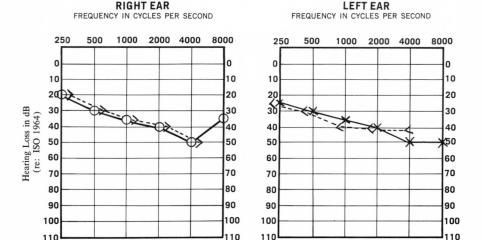

Figure 36 - Audiogram typical of patients with Alport's disease.
From Johnson, W.T. and Hagan, P.J., *Arch. Otolaryng.* 1965. Reproduced by permission.

to the effects of the drug for a longer time than usual. In these cases it may be impossible to ascertain whether the hearing loss is genetically determined or acquired. Therefore, any child with renal disease severe enough to warrant a renal transplant is included in the risk register, since the ototoxic effect of drugs administered may be enhanced by the renal disease.

B. *Endocrine Disorders*

    1. *Recessive hereditary disorders*

        a. Pendred's syndrome (10 percent of recessive hereditary deafness): Nonendemic goiter with onset in puberty with associated hypothyroidism, sensori-neural congenital deafness; vestibular function may be affected (see Figures 38A and 38B). Examination of the temporal bones of one patient showed Mondini-type pathology (Pendred 1896; Batsakis and Nishiyama 1962; DeCourt 1962; Fraser 1965b; Hvidberg-Hansen and Jorgensen 1968).

        b. Diabetes mellitus (juvenile) with associated optic atrophy and deafness. The deafness is of childhood, adolescent or early adult

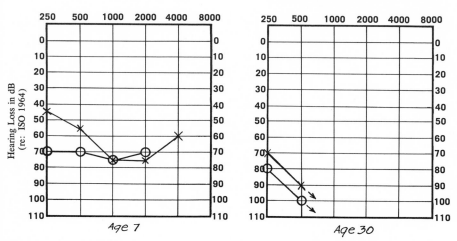

Figure 37 - Audiograms of a patient with urticaria and amyloidosis, showing progressing nature of loss over time.

Courtesy of Andersen et al. *Amer. J. Med.* 1967.

onset and is progressive. Audiogram may show only slight residual hearing but often only mild, high frequency loss is present (Shaw and Duncan 1959; Rose 1966).

2. *Dominant hereditary disorders*: None.

C. *Congenital Heart Disease*

    1. *Recessive hereditary disorders*

        a. Jervell and Lange-Nielsen's syndrome (1 percent of recessive hereditary deafness): Syncopal episodes due to heart disease and EKG abnormalities, early death, profound sensori-neural deafness (Jervell and Lange--Nielsen 1957; Levine and Woodworth 1958).

        b. Lewis' syndrome: Congenital pulmonary stenosis and sensori-neural deafness, apparently present since birth. Hypertelorism, generalized lentigines, and low-set ears are also seen (Lewis et al. 1958).

    2. *Dominant hereditary disorders*
Congenital heart disease, skeletal malformations and generalized lentigines. Conductive hearing loss is present due to congenital fixation of the stapes footplate (Forney et al. 1966).

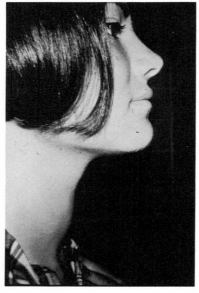

Figure 38A - Patient with Pendred's syndrome. Note the goiter. University of Colorado Medical Center

D. *Degenerative Disorders of the Nervous System* (Drachman 1968)

    1. *Recessive hereditary disorders*

        a. Friedreich's ataxia: Ataxia, loss of reflexes, nystagmus, optic atrophy, sensori-neural deafness. Onset, childhood. Temporal bone pathology: bilateral degeneration of the cochlear nerve and cochlear ganglion cells (Gates 1946; Nelson 1964).

        b. Unverricht's epilepsy: Myoclonic epilepsy, ataxia, dementia, partial to severe congenital "deafness" (Latham and Munro 1938).

        c. Cerebral palsy: Polyganglioradicular heredopathy and hypertrophic neuritis of Dejerine-Sottas. May have sensori-neural

[50]

loss, mild to severe (Kluyskens and Geldof 1965).

2. *Dominant hereditary disorders*

    a. Huntington's chorea: Degenerative chorea, dementia, either congenital or progressive "deafness," death. Onset at about age 35 (Nelson 1964; Gates 1946).

    b. Cerebellar ataxia, myoclonic seizures and sensori-neural hearing loss (May and White 1968).

    c. Hereditary photomyoclonus, diabetes mellitus, nephropathy,

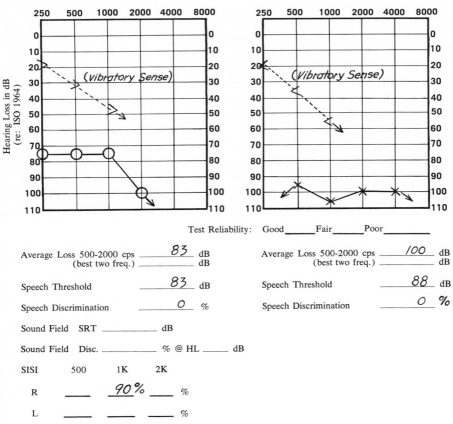

Figure 38B - Audiogram of 18-year-old girl with Pendred's syndrome. University of Colorado Medical Center

cerebral dysfunction and deafness. Onset in childhood or ado-
dolescence of light-sensitive seizures, later sensori-neural "deafness" of a progressive nature leading to severe impairment, high
SISI scores, type II Bekesy. Still later progressive dementia,
diabetes and low-grade pyelonephritis and glomerulonephritis.
PAS-positive lipid deposits are found in the brain (Herrmann
et al. 1964).

E. *Associated Brain Syndromes*
  1. *Recessive hereditary syndromes*
      a. Tay-Sach's disease: Amaurotic idiocy and "high-frequency
         deafness." Spasticity, seizures, dementia, death. Infant form
         appears at 6 months. Diagnosis by noting optic atrophy with
         macular cherry-red spots (Steinberg 1937; Jampel and Quaglio
         1964; Kelemen 1965b).
      b. Wilson's disease: Hepatolenticular degeneration affecting brain,
         liver and kidneys. Onset, age 5. Central nervous system symp-
         toms: dysarthria, tremor, seizures, dementia. Some "deafness"
         associated (Danish et al. 1963; Nelson 1964).
  2. *Dominant hereditary syndromes*
      Hereditary mental retardation with homocystinemia. Dislocated
      lenses, mild liver disease, severe retardation, "deafness" (Nelson
      1964).

F. *Other Neurologic Disorders*
  1. *Recessive hereditary syndromes*
      Severe infantile muscular dystrophy with deafness: Onset at birth
      of difficulty eating, later abnormal gait, facial weakness, eventually
      weakness of distal and proximal muscles, hypoactive tendon re-
      flexes (Schneck 1969). Sloping sensori-neural hearing loss of
      mild to moderate degree has been found by the authors (see Fig-
      ures 39A and 39B).
  2. *Dominant hereditary syndromes*
      Sensory radicular neuropathy and deafness: Painless ulceration of
      feet and progressive nerve deafness; both appear in early adult-
      hood and are progressive (Hicks 1922; Munro 1956). Temporal
      bone findings: severe degeneration of cochlear and vestibular
      hair cells with severe degenerative changes in stria vascularis,
      tectorial membrane and limbus. Cochlear nerve intact, but vesti-
      bular nerve degenerated (Denny-Brown 1951; Hallpike 1967).

G. *Hereditary Progressive Deafness Occurring Alone*
  1. *Recessive hereditary sensori-neural deafness:* May be congenital
      or progressive; hearing loss begins between the ages of 18 months

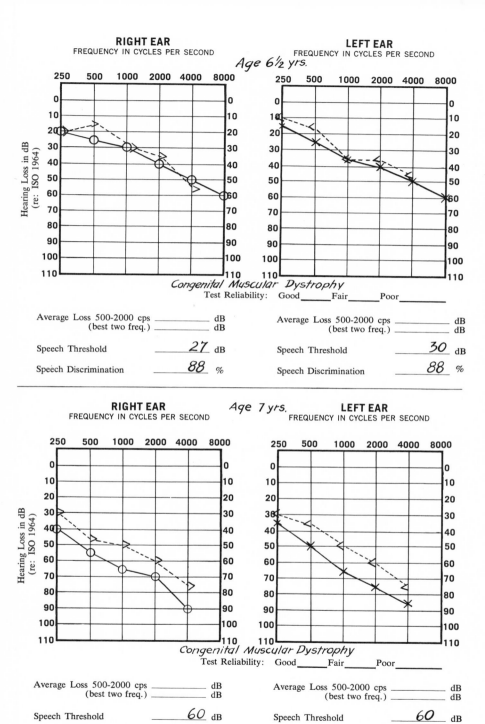

RIGHT EAR
FREQUENCY IN CYCLES PER SECOND

Age 6½ yrs.

LEFT EAR
FREQUENCY IN CYCLES PER SECOND

Congenital Muscular Dystrophy

Test Reliability: Good_____ Fair_____ Poor_____

Average Loss 500-2000 cps _____ dB
(best two freq.) _____ dB

Speech Threshold _____ *27* dB

Speech Discrimination _____ *88* %

Average Loss 500-2000 cps _____ dB
(best two freq.) _____ dB

Speech Threshold _____ *30* dB

Speech Discrimination _____ *88* %

RIGHT EAR
FREQUENCY IN CYCLES PER SECOND

Age 7 yrs.

LEFT EAR
FREQUENCY IN CYCLES PER SECOND

Congenital Muscular Dystrophy

Test Reliability: Good_____ Fair_____ Poor_____

Average Loss 500-2000 cps _____ dB
(best two freq.) _____ dB

Speech Threshold _____ *60* dB

Average Loss 500-2000 cps _____ dB
(best two freq.) _____ dB

Speech Threshold _____ *60* dB

Figures 39A & B - Audiograms of two children with severe congenital muscular dystrophy.
University of Colorado Medical Center

and 6 years, with progression to near total deafness by age 8 to 13. Audiometry typically shows a 75-100 dB loss in all frequencies. SISI scores are high (Fraser 1964; Mengel et al. 1967).

2. *Dominant hereditary sensori-neural deafness*: The most common audiometric pattern is either abrupt or gradually descending high-frequency loss. A degenerative change in the sensory and neural elements of the basal turn is present pathologically (Ersner and Saltzman 1941; Goodhill 1950; Johnson 1952; Cawthorne and Hinchcliffe 1957; Dolowitz and Stephens 1961). Unilateral deafness may also be a dominant hereditary trait. The onset may be delayed and sometimes shows a familial pattern of occurring after infections. The audiometric pattern varies from mild to total loss (Everberg 1960). The temporal bone pathology is Scheibe type with dilatation of the cochlear duct (Cohen et al. 1968). The importance of including this entity in a high risk register is to avoid in children at risk any possible other injury to the ears.

3. *Sex-linked hereditary sensori-neural deafness*: May be congenital and profound or progressive after childhood, or may involve only the high tones (Stephens and Dolowitz 1949; Sataloff et al. 1955; Mohr and Mageroy 1960; Livan 1961; Richards 1963; Fraser 1965a; McKusick 1968).

These are included in the occult classification because of confusion with acquired hearing losses.

III. Congenital Acquired Deafness of Prenatal, Perinatal and Neonatal Origin
   A. *Prenatal History*
      1. *History in family of deafness or other congenital abnormality*
      2. *Consanguinity* (Dolowitz and Stephens 1952; Feinmesser et al. 1966; Mengel et al. 1967; Brown 1967)
      3. *Rubella* or other virus diseases in first trimester or later in pregnancy (Eichenwald 1954; Baertschi 1966; Bordley et al. 1967; Alford 1968; Paparella and Winter 1968)
      4. *History of bleeding during pregnancy*
      5. *Ototoxic drugs taken during pregnancy.* Kanamycin, streptomycin, dihydrostreptomycin, viomycin, vancomycin, neomycin, terramycin, quinine, thalidomide, chloroquine (Kern 1962; Robinson and Cambon 1964; Podvinec et al. 1965; Hawkins 1967a and b; Matz and Naunton 1968).
      6. *History of toxemia during pregnancy*
      7. *Excessive x-ray exposure* during first trimester or even prior to pregnancy

8. *Rh incompatibility* with high anti-Rh titers in mother during pregnancy (Goodhill 1950, 1967)
9. *Diabetes in mother* (Strubinski and Malicka 1967)
10. *History of syphilis* (Perlman 1967)
11. *Toxoplasmosis* (Kelemen 1958)
12. *Nutritional defects*
13. *Anemia*
14. *Infections* (Hardy 1965)
15. *Immunizations*
16. *Cytomegalic inclusion disease* (Medearis 1964; Ward et al. 1965); Myers and Stool 1968)
17. *History of unexplained pre- or neonatal death* in previous pregnancy
18. *Maternal alcoholism or drug addiction*

B. *Perinatal History*
1. *Prolonged labor* — longer than 18 hours in primigravida, 8 hours in multigravida (Child 1968)
2. *Maternal hemorrhage,* abruptio placenta, placenta previa
3. *Infection*
4. *Ototoxic drugs* (Hawkins 1967a and b)
5. *Traction on neck,* forceps delivery, prolapsed cord, abnormal presentation
6. *Premature delivery* (Abramowicz and Kass 1966; Vernon 1967). Gestational age less than 36 weeks
7. *Fetal distress*: heart rate sustained at greater than 160/min. or less than 100/min. for 30 seconds; passage of meconium

C. *Neonatal History*
1. *Apnea or cyanosis* (Fisch 1955). Resuscitation requiring more than suctioning or simple stimulation (Child 1968)
2. *Jaundice-hyperbilirubinemia* — 15 mg/100cc and over or history of exchange transfusion (Goodhill 1950, 1967)
3. *Prolonged abnormality of central nervous system* (e.g. convulions)
4. *Paralysis*
5. *Prolonged stay in incubator*
6. *Abnormal birth weight* (Vernon 1967). Weight less than 1800 gms (4 lbs.) or over 5000 gms (11 lbs.)
7. *Discordant twins* (smaller twin 25 percent or more lighter than larger and weighing less than 2000 gms) (Child 1968)
8. *Ototoxic antibiotic used in treating infection in infant* (Marcus et al. 1963; Hawkins 1967 a and b). Ototoxic antibiotics are

more toxic in the infant with renal disease or decreased renal function, as in premature infants

9. *Hearing screening testing abnormal* (Downs and Sterritt 1967; Downs and Hemenway 1969)
10. *Any of symptoms described under overt symptomatology*

References

Abramowicz, M. and Kass, E.H. 1966. Pathogenesis and prognosis of prematurity. *New Eng. J. Med.* 275:938-43; 1001-7; 1053-59.

Alberti, P.W.R.M. and Parkannen, J.V. 1963. Stapedial otosclerosis: recent histochemical and histopathological observations. *Laryngoscope* 73:1184-1200.

Alexander, G. 1904. Zur Pathologie und pathologischen Anatomie der Kongenetalen Taubheit. *Arch. Ohr. Nas. Kehlkopfheilk* 61:183-219.

Alford, B.R. 1968. Rubella—la bête noire de la médecine. *Laryngoscope* 88:1623-59.

Alport, A.C. 1927. Hereditary familial congenital hemorrhagic nephritis. *Brit. Med. J.* 1:504-6.

Alstrom, C.H.; Hallgren, B.; Nilsson, L.B. and Asander, H. 1959. Retinal degeneration combined with obesity, diabetes mellitus and neurogenous deafness. *Acta Psychiat. Scand.* (Suppl. 34) 129:1-35.

Altmann, F. 1962. The temporal bone in osteogenesis imperfecta congenita. *Arch. Otolaryng.* 75:486-97.

————. 1968. Histologic findings in congenital deafness. *Acta Otolaryng.* 65:115-19.

Andersen, V.; Buch, N.H.; Jensen, M.K.; and Killmann, S. 1967. Deafness, urticaria and amyloidosis. *Amer. J. Med.* 42:449-56.

Anderson, H. and Wedenberg, E. 1968. Audiometric identification of normal hearing carriers of genes for deafness. *Acta Otolaryng.* 65:535-54.

Arthur, L.J.H. 1965. Some hereditary syndromes that include deafness. *Develop. Med. Child Neurol.* 7:395-409.

Baertschi, V. 1966. Rubella virus and embryopathies. *Bibl. Gynaec.* 39:1-59.

Bardadin, T. and Siedlanowska, H. 1955. Congenital deafness in Klippel-Feil's syndrome. *Otolaryng. Pol.* 9:25-31.

Bart, R.S. and Pumphrey, R.E. 1967. Knuckle pads, leukonychia and deafness. *New Eng. J. Med.* 276:202-7.

Batsakis, J.G. and Nishiyama, R.H. 1962. Deafness with sporadic goiter: Pendred's syndrome. *Arch. Otolaryng.* 76:401-6.

Beaney, G.P.E. 1964. Otolaryngological problems arising during the management of severe renal failure. *J. Laryng.* 78:507-15.

[57]

Black, F.O.; Sando, I.; Wagner, J.A.; and Hemenway, W.G. 1970. A 13-15 (D₁) trisomy with middle and inner ear abnormalities. In manuscript.

Bochenek, A. and Mitkiewicz-Szreniawska, W. 1958. Hearing examination in retinitis pigmentosa. *Otolaryng. Pol.* 12:456-63.

Bordley, J.E. and Hardy, W.G. 1951. Etiology of deafness in young children. *Acta Otolaryng.* 40:72-9.

Bordley, J.E.; Brookhouser, P.E.; Hardy, J.; and Hardy, W.G. 1967. Observations on the effect of prenatal rubella in hearing. Chapter 9, *Deafness in Childhood*, ed. McConnell, F. and Ward, P.H., pp. 123-41. Vanderbilt University Press.

Braun, F.C., Jr. and Bayer, J.F. 1962. Familial nephrosis associated with deafness and congenital urinary tract anomalies in siblings. *J. Pediat.* 60:33-41.

Brown, Kenneth S. 1967. The genetics of childhood deafness. Chapter 12, *Deafness in Childhood*, ed. McConnell, F. and Ward, P.H., pp. 177-202. Vanderbilt University Press.

Buran, D.J. and Duvall, A.J. 1967. The oto-palato-digital syndrome. *Arch. Otolaryng.* 85:394-99.

Burn, R.A. 1950. Deafness and Laurence-Moon-Biedl syndrome. *Brit. J. Ophthal.* 34:64-88.

Carhart, R. 1967. Audiologic tests: questions and speculations. Chapter 15, *Deafness in Childhood*, ed. McConnell, F. and Ward, P.H., pp. 229-51. Vanderbilt University Press.

Cawthorne, T.E. and Hinchcliffe, R. 1957. Familial perceptive deafness. *Pract. Otorhinolaryng.* 19:69-83.

Child, S. 1968. (Personal communication to authors) From *High Risk Questionnaire*, Div. of Maternal & Child Health; Dept. of Public Health, State of Utah, Salt Lake City.

Clerc, P. and Deumier, R. 1958. Deafness in osseous dysplasia and craniofacial dysmorphia. *Ann. Otol.* Paris, 74:852-74.

Cody, T. and Williams, H. 1960. Cogan's syndrome. *Laryngoscope* 70:447-78.

Cogan, D.G. 1945. Syndrome of non-syphilitic interstitial keratitis and vestibulo-auditory symptoms. *Arch. Ophthal.* 33:144-49.

Cohen, M.M.; Cassady, G. and Hanna, B.L. 1961. A genetic study of hereditary renal dysfunction with associated nerve deafness. *Amer. J. Human Genetics* 13:379-89.

Cohn, A.M.; Beal, D.D. and Kohut, R.I. 1968. Inner ear pathology in unilateral congenital deafness. *Ann. Otol. Rhinol. & Laryngol.* 77:43-53.

Crouzon, O. 1912. Dysostose cranio faciale hereditaire. *Bull. Soc. Med. Hôp. Paris.* 33:545-55.

Cushing, H. 1916. Hereditary ankylosis of the proximal interphalangeal joints. *Genetics* 1:90-106.

Danish, J.M.; Tillson, J.K.; and Levitan, M. 1963. Multiple anomalies in congenitally deaf children. *Eugen. Quart.* 10:12-21.

d'Avignon, M. and Barr, B. 1964. Ear abnormalities and cranial nerve palsies in Thalidomide children. *Arch. Otolaryng.* 80:136-40.

DeCourt, J. 1962. Study of three cases of goiter with deaf-mutism in a single family (Pendred's syndrome). *Ann. Endocr.* 23:381-93.

Denny-Brown, D. 1951. Hereditary sensory radicular neuropathy. *J. Neurol. Neurosurg. & Psychiat.* 14:237-52.

DeVos, J.A. 1963. Deafness in hypothyroidism. *J. Laryng.* 77:390-414.

DiGeorge, A.M.; Olmstead, R.W.; and Harley, R.D. 1960. Waardenburg's syndrome. *J. Pediat.* 57:649-69.

Dolowitz, D.A. and Stephens, F.E. 1961. Hereditary nerve deafness. *Ann. Otol., Rhinol. & Laryngol.* 70:851-59.

Dolowitz, D.A. and Stephens, F.E. 1952. Hereditary progressive nerve deafness. *Trans. Amer. Acad. Ophthal. Otolaryng.* 56:457-64.

Downs, M.P. and Sterritt, G.M. 1967. A guide to newborn and infant hearing screening programs. *Arch. Otolaryng.* 85:15-22.

Downs, M.P. 1969. *Organization and procedures of a newborn infant screening program.* Official Publication of the Nat'l. Assn. of Hearing and Sp. Agencies, Wash. D.C.

Downs, M.P. and Hemenway, W.G. 1969. Report on the hearing screening of 17,000 neonates. *Int'l. Audiology* 8:72-76.

Drachman, D.A. 1968. Ophthalmoplegia plus. *Arch. Neurol.* 18:654-74.

Ebihara, I.; Takayasu, S.; and Ikeda, H. 1959. A rare case of Heerfordt's disease complicated by bilateral perceptive deafness. *Oto-Rhino-Laryng. Soc. Japan* 62:1568-72.

Eichenwald, H.G. 1954. The placental "barrier" and infections of the fetus. *J.Laryng.* 68:329-30.

Ersner, M.S. and Saltzman, M. 1941. Progressive analogous nerve deafness in three successive generations with sex-limited inheritance. *Laryngoscope* 51:241-45.

Everberg, G. 1960. Further studies on hereditary unilateral deafness. *Acta Otolaryng.* 51:615-35.

————. 1959. Marfan's syndrome associated with hearing defect: report of a case in one of a pair of twins. *Acta Paediat.* 48:70-76.

Feinmesser, M. and Zelig, S. 1961. Congenital deafness associated with onychodystrophy. *Arch. Otolaryng.* 74:507-8.

Feinmesser, M.; Bauberger-Tell, L.; and Markus, F. 1966. Consanguinity among parents of deaf children in the Jewish population in Israel. *J. Laryng.* 80:1253-56.

[59]

Fernandez, A.O. and Ronis, M.L. 1964. The Treacher Collins syndrome. *Arch. Otolaryng.* 80:505-20.

Fickentscher, H. 1954. Klippel-Feil syndrome and hardness of hearing. *Arch. Ohr. Nas. Kehlkopfheilk* 164:297-307.

Fisch, L. 1959. Deafness as part of an hereditary syndrome. *J. Laryng.* 73:355-82.

————. 1955. The aetiology of congenital deafness and audiometric patterns. *J. Laryng.* 69:479-93.

Forney, W.R.; Robinson, S.J.; and Pascoe, D.J. 1966. Congenital heart disease, deafness and skeletal malformations: a new syndrome? *J. Ped.* 68:14-19.

Fourman, P. and Fourman, J. 1955. Hereditary deafness in a family with ear-pits. *Brit. Med. J.* 2:1354-56.

Francois, J. 1961. *Heredity in Ophthalmology.* St. Louis: The C.V. Mosby Co.

Fraser, G.R. 1964. Review article, Profound childhood deafness, *J. Med. Genetics* 1:118-51.

————. 1965a. Sex-linked recessive congenital deafness and the excess of males in profound childhood deafness. *Ann. Hum. Genet.* 29:171-96.

————. 1965b. Association of congenital deafness with goitre (Pendred's syndrome). *Ann. Hum. Genet.* 28:201-49.

Fraser, J.S. 1926-27. A case of congenital deafness with malformation of the membranous labyrinths of both sides. *Proc. Roy. Soc. Med.* (Sect. Otol.) 20:17-19.

Friedmann, I.; Fraser, G.R. and Froggatt, P. 1965. The pathology of the ear in the cardioauditory syndrome of Jervell and Lange-Nielsen (recessive deafness with electrocardiographic abnormalities). *J. Laryng.* 80:451-69.

Gardner, W.J. and Turner O. 1940. Bilateral acoustic neurofibromas. *Arch. Neurol. Psychiat.* 44:76-99.

Gates, R. 1946. *Human Genetics.* New York: The Macmillan Co.

Gerich, J.E. 1969. Hunter's syndrome: Beta-galactosidase deficiency in skin. *New Eng. J. Med.* 280:799-801.

Globus, J.H. and Strauss, I. 1928. Progressive degenerative subcortical encephalopathy (Schilder's disease). *Arch. Neurol. Psychiat.* 20:1190-1228.

Goldbloom, R.B.; Fraser, F.C.; Waugh, D.; Aronovitch, M. and Wiglesworth, F.W. 1957. Hereditary renal disease and ocular lesions. *Pediatrics* 20:241-52.

Goldman, R. and Haberfelde, G.C. 1959. Hereditary nephritis: report of a kindred. *New Eng. J. Med.* 261:734-38.

Goodhill, V. 1939. Syphilis of the ear: a histopathologic study. *Ann. Otol., Rhinol. & Laryng.* 48:676-706.

————. 1950. The nerve-deaf child: significance of Rh, maternal rubella and other etiologic factors. *Ann. Otol., Rhinol. & Laryng..* 59:1123-47.

————. 1967. Auditory pathway lesions resulting from Rh incompatibility. Chapter 14, *Deafness in Childhood,* ed. McConnell, F. and Ward, P.H. pp. 215-28. Vanderbilt University Press.

Gorlin, R.J. and Pindborg, J.J. 1964. *Syndromes of the Head and Neck.* New York: McGraw-Hill, pp. 138-45.

Goyer, R.A.; Reynolds, J.; Burke, J.; and Burkholder, P. 1968. Hereditary renal disease with neurosensory hearing loss, prolinuria and ichthyosis. *Amer. J. Med. Sci.* 256:166-79.

Greiner, G.F.; Brini, A.; and Grossmann, M. 1962. The association of late deafness and retinitis pigmentosa. *Rev. Oto-Neuro-Ophthal.* 34:54-58.

Guilford, F.R. 1967. Surgical treatment of hearing losses in children. Chapter 13, *Deafness in Childhood,* ed. McConnell, F. and Ward, P.H. pp. 203-14. Vanderbilt University Press.

Hall, J.G. and Rφhrt, T. 1968. The stapes in osteogenesis imperfecta. *Acta Otolaryng.* 65:345-48.

Hallgren, B. 1959. Retinitis pigmentosa combined with congenital deafness, with vestibulo-cerebellar ataxia and mental abnormality in a proportion of cases. *Acta Psychiat. Scand.* (Suppl. 34) 138:1-101.

Hall-Jones, J. 1963. Congenital deafness. *New Zeal. Med. J.* 62:470-75.

Hallpike, C.S. 1967. Observations on the structural basis of two rare varieties of hereditary deafness, in *Myotactic Kinesthetic and Vestibular Mechanisms* (Ciba Foundation Symposium), ed. DeReuck, A.V.S., Boston: Little, Brown & Co.

Hamburger, J.; Crosnier, J.; Lissae, J.; and Naffah, J. 1956. Sur un syndrome familial de nephropathie avec surdité. *J. Urol.* (*Paris*) 62:113-24.

Hardy, J.B. 1965. Viral infections in pregnancy: a review. *Amer. J. Ob. Gyn.* 93:1052-65.

Hawkins, J.E., Jr. 1967a. Iatrogenic toxic deafness in children. Chapter 11, *Deafness in Childhood,* ed. McConnell, F. and Ward, P.H. pp. 156-68. Vanderbilt University Press.

————. 1967b. Antibiotic insults to Corti's organ, in *Sensorineural Hearing Processes and Disorders,* ed. Graham, G. Boston: Little, Brown & Co.

Helweg-Larsen, H.F. and Ludvigsen, K. 1946. Congenital familial anhidrosis and neurolabyrinthitis. *Acta Dermatovener* 26:489-505.

Hemenway, W.G. and Bergstrom, L. 1967. The pathology of acquired viral endolabyrinthitis. Chapter 8, *Deafness in Childhood,* ed. McConnell, F. and Ward, P.H., pp. 91-122, Vanderbilt University Press.

Hemenway, W.G.; Sando, I.; and McChesney, D. 1969. Temporal bone pathology following maternal rubella. *Arch. für klinische u. exper. Ohr.-Nas.-u. Kehlkopfheilk.* 193:287-300.

Herrmann, C., Jr.; Aguilar, M.J. and Sacks, O.W. 1964. Hereditary photo-myoclonus associated with diabetes mellitus, deafness, nephropathy, and cerebral dysfunction. *Neurology* 14:212-21.

Hicks, E.P. 1922. Hereditary perforating ulcer of the foot. *Lancet* 1:319-21.

Hough, J.V.D. 1958. Malformations and anatomical variations seen in the middle ear during the operation for mobilization of the stapes. *Laryngoscope* 68:1337-78.

Howarth, A.S. and Lloyd, H.E.D. 1956. Perceptive deafness in hypothyroidism. *Brit. Med. J.* 1:431-32.

Hunter, C. 1917. A rare disease in two brothers. *Proc. Roy. Soc. Med.* 10:104-16.

Hurler, G. 1919. Ueber einen Typ Multipler Abartgungen, vorwiegend am Skelett-system. *Ztsch. Kinderh.* 24:220-34.

Hvidberg-Hansen J. and Jorgensen, M.B. 1968. The inner ear in Pendred's syndrome. *Acta Otolaryng.* 66:129-35.

Jampel, R.S. and Quaglio, N.D. 1964. Eye movements in Tay-Sachs disease. *Neurology* 14:1013-19.

Jervell, A. and Lange-Nielsen, F. 1957. Congenital deaf-mutism, functional heart disease with prolongation of the QT interval and sudden death. *Amer. Heart J.* 54:59-68.

Johnson, S. 1952. The heredity of perceptive deafness. *Acta Otolaryng.* 42:539-52.

Johnson, W.T. and Hagan, P.J. 1965. Hereditary nephropathy and loss of hearing. *Arch. Otolaryng.* 82:166-72.

Jorgensen, M.B. and Kristensen, H.K. 1964. Thalidomide induced aplasia of the inner ear. *J. Laryng.* 78:1095-1101.

Karmody, C.S. and Schuknecht, H.F. 1966. Deafness in congenital syphilis. *Arch. Otolaryng.* 83:18-26.

Kelemen, G. 1965a. Marfan's syndrome and the hearing organ. *Acta Otolaryng.* 59:23-32.

————. 1966a. Rubella and deafness. *Arch. Otolaryng.* 83:520-32.

————. 1965b. Tay-Sachs-Krankheit und Gehororgan. Z. *Laryng. Rhin. Otol.* 44:729-38.

————. 1958. Toxoplasmosis and congenital deafness. *Arch. Otolaryng.* 68:547-61.

————. 1966b. Hurler's syndrome and the hearing organ. *J. Laryng.* 80:791-803.

Kern, G. 1962. Zur Frage der Intrauterinen streptomycinschadigung. *Schweiz. Med. Wschr.* 92:77-79.

Klintworth, G.K. 1963. Neurological manifestations of osteopetrosis (Albers-Schonberg's disease). *Neurology* 13:512-19.

Kluyskens, P. and Geldof, H. 1965. La surdité hereditaire. *Acta Oto-rhino-laryng. Belg.* 19:519-43.

Kos, A.O.; Schuknecht, H.F. and Singer, J.D. 1966. Temporal bone studies in 13-15 & 18 trisomy syndromes. *Arch. Otolaryng.* 83:439-55.

Latham, A.D. and Munro, T.A. 1938. Familial myoclonus epilepsy associated with deaf-mutism in a family showing other psychobiological abnormalities. *Ann. Eugen.* 8:166-75.

Laurence, K.M. 1964. Arhinencephaly and trisomy of the 13-15 chromosomes. *Arch. Dis. Child.* 39:302-3.

Levine, S.A. and Woodworth, C.R. 1958. Congenital deaf-mutism, prolonged QT interval, syncopal attacks and sudden death. *New Eng. J. Med.* 259:412-17.

Lewis, S.M.; Sonnenblick, B.P.; Gilbert, L. and Biber, D. 1958. Familial pulmonary stenosis and deaf-mutism: clinical and genetic considerations. *Amer. Heart J.* 55:458-62.

Lichtenstein, B.W. and Rosenbluth, P.P. 1956. Schilder's disease with melanoderma. *J. Neur. Path. & Exp. Neurology* 15:229-31.

Lindeman, R.C. 1967. Congenital sensorineural deafness, in *Sensorineural Hearing Processes and Disorders,* ed. Graham, B., Boston: Little, Brown & Co.

Lindsay, J.R. 1967. Labyrinthitis of viral origin, in *Sensorineural Hearing Processes and Disorders,* ed. Graham, B., Boston: Little, Brown & Co.

Livan, M. 1961. Contribute alla conscenza della sorbita ereditarie. *Arch. Ital. Otol.* 72:331-39.

Livingstone, G. and Delahunty, J.E. 1968. Malformation of the ear associated with congenital ophthalmic and other conditions. *J. Laryng.* 82:495-504.

Ludman, H.; Hamilton, E.B.D. and Eade, A.W.T. 1968. Deafness in myositis ossificans progressiva. *J. Laryng.* 82:57-63.

McKenzie, J. 1958. The first arch syndrome. *Arch. Dis. Child.* 33:477-86.

McKusick, V.A. 1960. Medical genetics, 1959. *J. Chronic Dis.* 12:129-32.

————. 1968. *Mendelian Inheritance in Man.* ed. 2. Baltimore: Johns Hopkins Press.

————. 1966. *Heritable Disorders of Connective Tissue,* ed. 3. St. Louis: C.V. Mosby Co.

McLaurin, J.W.; Kloepfer, H.W.; Laguaite, J.K.; and Stallcup, T.A. 1966. Hereditary branchial anomalies and associated hearing impairment. *Laryngoscope* 76:1277-88.

McLay, K. and Maran, A.G.D. 1969. Deafness and the Klippel-Feil syndrome. *J. Laryng.* 83:175-84.

Maran, A.G.D. 1964. The Treacher Collins syndrome. *J. Laryng.* 78:135-51.

Marcus, R.E.; Small, H. and Emanuel, B. 1963. Ototoxic medication in premature children. *Arch Otolaryng.* 77:198-204.

————. 1968. Vestibular function and additional findings in Waardenburg's syndrome. *Acta Otol. Suppl.* 229:5-30.

Margolis, E. 1962. A new hereditary syndrome—sex-linked deafmutism associated with total albinism. *Acta Genet. Statist. Med.* 12:12-19.

Marshall, D. 1958. Ectodermal dysplasia: report of kindred with ocular abnormalities and hearing defect. *Amer. J. Ophthal.* 45:143-56.

Matz, G.J. and Naunton, R.F. 1968. Ototoxicity of Chloroquine. *Arch. Otolaryng.* 88:370-72.

May, D.L. and White, H.H. 1968. Familial myoclonus, cerebellar ataxia and deafness. *Arch. Neurol.* 19:331-38.

Mayer, O. and Fraser, J.S. 1936. Pathological changes in the ear in late congenital syphilis. *J. Laryng.* 51:683-714.

Medearis, D.N., Jr. 1964. Observations concerning human cytomegalovirus infection and disease. *Bull. Johns Hopkins Hosp.* 114:181-211.

Mendelsohn, R.S. and Cohen, B. 1964. Otorhinolaryngologic aspects of cystic fibrosis. *Arch. Otolaryng.* 79:312-17.

Mengel, M.C.; Konigsmark, B.W.; Berlin, C.I.; and McKusick, V.A. 1967. Recessive early-onset neural deafness. *Acta Otolaryng.* 64:313-26.

Mengel, M.C.; Konigsmark, B.W.; Berlin, C.I.; and McKusick, V.A. 1969. Familial conductive hearing loss and malformed, low-set ears, probably a new entity. *J. Med. Genetics* 6:14-21.

Michel, E.M. 1863. Memoire sur les anomalies congenitales de l'oreille interne. *Gaz. Med. Strasb.* 3:55-58.

Miller, J.Q.; Picard, E.H.; Alkan, M.K.; Warner, S. and Gerald, P.S. 1963. A specific congenital brain defect (Arhinencephaly) in 13-15 trisomy. *New Eng. J. Med.* 268:120-23.

Mohr, J. and Mageroy, K. 1960. Sex-linked deafness of a possibly new type. *Acta Genet. Statist. Med.* 10:54-62.

Mondini, C. 1791. Anatomia surdi nedi sectio, *DeBononiensi Scientarium et Artium Instituto Atque Academi Commentarii,* Bologna, 7:28-29, 419-31.

Moro, F. and Amidei, B. 1957. Spotted dystrophy or Fehr's dystrophy of the cornea with deafness and stammering. *Ann. Otol.* 83:30-52.

Muckle, T.J. and Wells, M. 1962. Urticaria, deafness and amyloidosis: a new heredo-familial syndrome. *Quart. J. Med.* 31:235-48.

Munro, M. 1956. Sensory radicular neuropathy in a deaf child. *Brit. Med. J.* 1:541-44.

Myers, E.N. and Stool, S. 1968. Cytomegalic inclusion disease of the inner ear. *Laryngoscope* 78:1904-15.

Nakamura, S. and Sando I. 1966. Congenital absence of the oval window. *Arch. Otolaryng.* 84:131-36.

Nath, K.; Vijay, S.D.; Nema, H.V. and Shukla, B.R. 1964. Crouzon's disease and pituitary dysfunction. *Brit. J. Ophthal.* 48:162-164.

Naunton, R.F. and Valvassori, G.E. 1968. Inner ear anomalies: their association with atresia. *Laryngoscope* 78:1041-49.

Nelson, W.E. ed. 1964. *Textbook of Pediatrics,* ed. 8. Philadelphia: W.B. Saunders Co.

Opheim, O. 1968. Loss of hearing following the syndrome of Van Der Hoeve-de Kleyn, *Acta Otolaryng.,* 65:337-44.

Paddison, R.M.; Moossy, J.; and Derbes, V.J. 1963. Cockayne's syndrome. *Derm. Trop.* 2:195-203.

Paparella, M.M. and Winter, L.E. 1968. Sensori-neural deafness in childhood. *Trans. Amer. Acad. Ophthal. Otolaryng.* 72:782-88.

Paparella, M.M. and Suguira, S. 1967. The pathology of suppurative labyrinthitis. *Ann. Otol, Rhinol, and Laryngol.* 76:554-86.

Paparella, M.M. 1969. Sensorineural deafness in children. Paper delivered at Medical Audiology Workshop, Vail, Colorado.

Patau, K.; Smith, D.W.; Therman, E.; Inhorn, S.L. and Wagner, H.P. 1960. Multiple congenital anomaly caused by an extra autosome. *Lancet* 1:790-93.

Pendred, V. 1896. Deaf mutism and goitre. *Lancet* 2:532.

Perkoff, G.T. 1967. The hereditary renal diseases. *New Eng. J. Med.* 277:79-85, 129-38.

Perlman, H.B. 1967. Some labyrinth capsule diseases and inner ear deafness, in *Sensorineural Hearing Processes and Disorders,* ed. Graham, B. Boston: Little, Brown & Co.

Perlman, H.B. and Leek, J.H. 1952. Late congenital syphilis of the ear. *Laryngoscope* 62:1175-96.

Podvinec, B.M.; Marcetic, A. and Simonovic, M. 1965. Schadigungen des fotalen Cortischen Organs durch Streptomycin. *Monatschrift für Ohren Heilk und Laryngo-Rhino.* 99:20-24.

Pou, J.W. 1963. Congenital absence of the oval window. *Laryngoscope* 73:384-91.

Proctor, C.A. and Proctor, B. 1967. Understanding hereditary nerve deafness. *Arch. Otolaryng.* 85:23-40.

Refsum, S. 1946. Heredopathia Atactica Polyneuritiformis. *Acta Psychiat. Scand. (Suppl)* 38:1-303.

————. 1954. Heredoataxia hemeralopia polyneuritiformis—et tidligere ikke beskrevet familiaert syndrom? *Nord. Med.* 28:2682-85.

Reisman, L.E. and Matheny, A.P., Jr. 1969. *Genetics and Counseling in Medical Practice.* St. Louis: C.V. Mosby Co.

Remky, H.; Klier, A.; and Kober, J. 1964-65. Macular dystrophy with deaf-mutism in: *The Year Book of the Ear, Nose, and Throat*, J.R. Lindsay ed. Chicago: Year Book Medical Publishers, Inc. 1964-1965 series, pp. 59-60.

Richards, B.W. 1963. Sex-linked deaf-mutism. *Ann. Hum. Genet.* 26:195-99.

Richards, B.W. and Rundle, A.T. 1959. A familial hormonal disorder associated with neural deficiency, deaf-mutism and ataxia. *J. Ment. Deficiency Research* 3:33-55.

Richards, C.S. 1964. Middle ear changes in rubella deafness. *Arch. Otolaryng.* 80:48-59.

Robinson, G.C. and Johnston, M.M. 1967. Pili torti and sensory neural hearing loss. *J. Pediat.* 70:621-23.

Robinson, G.C.; Miller, J.R. and Bensimon, J.R. 1962. Familial ectodermal dysplasia with sensori-neural deafness and other anomalies. *Pediatrics* 30:797-802.

Robinson, G.D. and Cambon, K.G. 1964. Hearing loss in infants of tuberculous mothers treated with streptomycin during pregnancy. *New Eng. J. Med.* 271:949-51.

Rose, F.C.; Fraser, G.R.; and Friedmann, A.I. 1966. The association of juvenile diabetes mellitus and optic atrophy: clinical and genetical aspects. *Quart. J. Med.* 35:385-405.

Rosenberg, A.L.; Bergstrom, L.; Troost, B.T. and Bartholomew, B. 1970. Hyperuricemia and neurologic deficits—a family study. *New Eng. J. Med.* 282:992-97.

Sacrez, R.; Francfort, J.J.; and Gigonnet, J.M. 1967. Concerning the mental retardation and anomalies associated with the symptomatic triad of the Pierre Robin syndrome. *Ann. Pediat.* Paris, 14:28-33.

Sando, I.; Hemenway, W.G.; and Morgan, W.R. 1968. Histopathology of the temporal bones in mandibulo-facial dysostosis (Treacher Collins syndrome). *Trans. Amer. Acad. Ophthal., Otolaryng.* 72:913-24.

Sando, I.; Bergstrom, L.; Wood, R.P., and Hemenway, W.G. 1970. Temporal bone findings in trisomy 18 syndrome. *Arch. Otolaryng.* 91:552-59.

Sataloff, J.; Pastore, P.N.; and Bloom, E. 1955. Sex-linked hereditary deafness. *Amer. J. Hum. Genet.* 7:201-3.

Schafer, I.A.; Scriver, C.R.; and Efron, M.L. 1962. Familial hyperprolinemia, cerebral dysfunction and renal anomalies occurring in a family with hereditary nephropathy and deafness. *New Eng. J. Med.* 267:51-60.

Scheibe, A. 1892. A case of deaf-mutism, birth auditory atrophy and anomalies of development in the membranous labyrinth of both ears. *Arch. Otol.* 21:12-22.

Schilling, V. 1936. Striae distensae als hypophysaris Symptom bei basophilen

Vorder lappenadenom und bei Arachnodaktylie mit Hypophysentumor. *Med. Welt.* 10 (Feb. 8) 183; 10 (Feb. 15) 219; 10 (Feb. 22) 259.

Schneck, S. 1969. University of Colorado Medical Center, Denver, Colorado. Personal communication.

Schuknecht, H.F. 1967. Pathology of sensori-neural deafness of genetic origin. Chapter 7 in *Deafness in Childhood,* ed. McConnell, F. and Ward, P.H., pp. 69-90, Vanderbilt University Press.

Shaw, D.A. and Duncan, L.J.P. 1959. Optic atrophy and nerve deafness in diabetes mellitus. *J. Neurol. Neurosurg. Psychiat.* 21:47-49.

Shaw, R. and Glover, R. 1961. Abnormal segregation in hereditary renal diseases with deafness. *Amer. J. Hum. Genet.* 13:89-97.

Siebenmann, F. and Bing, R. 1907. Ueber den Labyrinth—und Hirnbefund bei einem an Retinitis pigmentosa erblindeten angelboren-taubstummen. *Z. Ohrenheilk* 54:265-80.

Singh, S.P.; Rock, E.H. and Shulman, A. 1969. Klippel-Feil syndrome with unexplained apparent conductive hearing loss. A case report. *Laryngoscope* 79:113-17.

Singleton, G.T. 1968. The alterations in hearing and histopathologic changes in Hurler's syndrome. Symposium Hearing Disorders in Children, Jan. 18-19, University of Oklahoma.

Steinberg, H. 1937. Erbliche Augenkrankheiten und Ohrenleiden. *Arch. Ohr. Nas. Kehlkopfheilk* 42:320-45.

Stephens, F.E. and Dolowitz, D.A. 1949. Hereditary nerve deafness. *Amer. J. Hum. Genet.* 1:37-51.

Strasburger, A.K.; Hawkins, M.R.; Eldridge, R.; Hargrave, R.L. and McKusick, V.A. 1965. Symphalangism: genetic and clinical aspects. *Bull. Johns Hopkins Hosp.* 117:108-27.

Strubinski, A. and Malicka, K. 1967. Localization of changes in the organ of hearing in diabetes. *Excerpta Medica* 20:100.

Szpunar, J. and Rybak, M. 1968. Middle ear disease in Turner's syndrome. *Arch. Otolaryng.* 87:34-40.

Tabor, J.R. 1961. Absence of the oval window. *Arch Otolaryng.* 74:515-21.

Taylor, W.C. 1965. Deformity of ears and kidneys. *Canad. Med. Assn. J.* 93:107-10.

Tietz, W. 1963. A syndrome of deaf-mutism associated with albinism showing dominant autosomal inheritance. *Amer. J. Hum. Genet.* 15:259-64.

Usher, C.H. 1914. On the inheritance of retinitis pigmentosum with notes of cases. *Roy. Lond. Ophthal. Hosp. Rep.* 19:130-236.

Vernon, M. 1967. Prematurity and deafness: the magnitude of the problem among deaf children. *Except. Child.* 33/5:289-98.

Von Graefe, A. 1858. Vereinzelte Beobachtungen und Bemerkungen No. 6

Exceptionelles Verhalten des Gesichtsfeldes bei Pigmententartung der Netz-haut, Graefe. *Arch. Ophthal.* 4:250-53.

Waardenburg, P.J. 1951. A new syndrome combining developmental anomalies of the eyelids, eyebrows and nose root with pigmentary defects of the iris and head hair and with congenital deafness. *Amer. J. Hum. Genet.* 3:195-253.

Wallenborn, P.A., Jr. 1960. Agammaglobulinemia, report of two cases and review of literature. *Laryngoscope* 70:1-36.

Warburg, M. 1963. Norrie's disease (atrofia bulborum hereditaria). *Acta Ophthal.* 41:134-46.

Ward, P.H.; Lindsay, J.R. and Warner, N.E. 1965. Cytomegalic inclusion disease affecting the temporal bone. *Laryngoscope* 75:628-36.

Warkany, J.; Passarge, E.; and Smith, L.B. 1966. Congenital malformation in autosomal trisomy syndromes. *Amer. J. Dis. Child.* 112 (6): 502-17.

Wildervanck, L.S. 1952. Een geval van aandoening van Klippel-Feil gecom-bineerd met abducens paralyse, retractio bulbi en doofstomheid. *Ned. T. Geneesk.* 96:2752.

Wildervanck, L.S.; Hoeksema, P.E.; and Penning, L. 1966. Radiological ex-amination of the inner ear of deaf-mutes presenting the cervico-oculo-acusti-cus syndrome. *Acta Otolaryng.* 61:445-53.

Wolff, C.M.; Dolowitz, D.A.; and Aldous, H.E. 1965. Congenital deafness associated with piebaldness. *Arch. Otolaryng.* 82:244-50.

Wolff, D. 1942. Microscopic study of temporal bones in dysostosis multiplex (gargoylism). *Laryngoscope* 52:218-23.

Wolff, D.; Bernhard, W.G.; Tsutsumi, S.; Ross, I.S.; and Nussbaum, H.E. 1965. The pathology of Cogan's syndrome causing profound deafness. *Ann. Otol. Rhinol., and Laryngol.* 74:507-20.

Yarington, C.T. and Sprinkle, P. 1967. Hearing problems in certain forms of osteodystrophy. The chondrodystrophies. *The Eye, Ear, Nose and Throat Monthly.* 46:1136-38.

Zellweger, H. 1965. Chromosomal aberrations and their significance for oph-thalmo-otorhinolaryngology. *Trans. Amer. Acad. Ophthal. Otolaryng.* 69:33-50.

Ziprkowski, L. and Adam A. 1964. Recessive total albinism and congenital deafmutism. *Arch. Derm.* 89:151-55.

DIVISION OF OTOLARYNGOLOGY
AND AUDIOLOGY SECTION
UNIVERSITY OF COLORADO MEDICAL CENTER

HIGH RISK CHECK LIST

Definition: High Risk Infant (Hearing Loss): An infant is suspect for hearing loss who has a history or condition which may be concomitant with hearing impairment.

Baby's Name ....
Birth Date ....
Mother's Name ....
Father's or Guardian's Name ....
Home Address ....
Physician ....
Hospital ....
City .... County ....

Item No.	Instructions: This check list may be completed by reference to (1) Mother's chart, (2) Infant's chart, (3) Direct observation of infant.	Yes	No	Unknown

I. *Prenatal Conditions*

1. Family history of deafness or other congenital abnormality.
2. Consanguinity.
3. Rubella or other virus disease during pregnancy.
4. Any bleeding indicating threatened abortion during pregnancy.
5. Ototoxic drugs taken during pregnancy. Kanamycin, streptomycin, dihydrostreptomycin, viomycin, neomycin, terramycin, quinine, thalidomide, chloroquine.
6. Toxemia of pregnancy—eclampsia and pre-eclampsia.
7. Excessive radiation exposure during pregnancy.
8. Rh incompatibility with rising anti-Rh titers during pregnancy.
9. Concurrent maternal diabetes.
10. Concurrent maternal syphilis.
11. Concurrent maternal toxoplasmosis.
12. Concurrent maternal malnutrition sufficient to be of clinical concern.

[69]

13. Concurrent maternal anemia sufficient to be of clinical concern.
14. Concurrent serious maternal acute infection.
15. Immunizations.
16. Cytomegalic inclusion disease.
17. History of previous unexplained pre- or neonatal death.
18. Maternal alcoholism or drug addiction.

II. *Perinatal Conditions*

1. Prolonged labor: longer than 18 hours in primigravida, 8 hours in multigravida.
2. Precipitate or uncontrolled delivery.
3. Maternal hemorrhage, abruptio placenta, placenta previa.
4. Sepsis or other infection present.
5. Traction on neck, high or mid-forceps delivery, prolapsed cord, abnormal presentation, version and extraction.
6. Gestational age under 36 weeks or over 42 weeks.
7. Fetal distress: heart rate sustained at greater than 160/min. or less than 100/min. for 30 seconds; passage of meconium.

III. *Neonatal Conditions*

1. Apnea or cyanosis. Resuscitation requiring more than suctioning or simple stimulation.
2. Ototoxic drug used in treating infection in infant.
3. Jaundice-hyperbilirubinemia: 15mg/100 cc and over; a history of exchange transfusions.
4. Prolonged abnormality of central nervous systey, e.g. convulsions.
5. Paralysis.
6. Birth weight less than 1800 gms (4 lbs.) or over 5000 gms (11 lbs.).
7. Discordant twin (smaller twin 25% or more

lighter and weighing less than 2000 gms at birth.)

8. Hearing Screening Test abnormal.

9. Any of the following observed conditions:

a. Skeletal and cranial defects: skull abnormalities........, short neck........, absent clavicles ...., dwarfism........, malformations of extremities and digits........, cleft lip........, cleft palate (overt or submucous)........, underdeveloped maxillae or mandible........, facial asymmetry (including facial paralysis)........, external ear abnormalities........, low hairline ...., fragile bones associated with blue sclerae........, knuckle pads........, white nails ....

b. Eye abnormalities: blindness........, chorioretinitis........, retinal and corneal abnormalities ...., optic atrophy........, small sunken eyes ...., cataracts........, colobomata (clefts) of eyelids or of iris........, ocular palsy or paralysis........, anti-mongoloid slant of eyes........, dislocated lenses.........

c. Pigmentary abnormalities: unusually light skin........, absence of skin appendages........, lack of pigment in iris........, sclera and fundus ...., abnormal canthi........, white forelock ...., different colored irises........, wide root of nose........, wide separation of eyes........, clumps of pigment in retina........, generalized lentigines.........

d. Associated ectodermal abnormalities: Any unusual condition of: hair........, nails........, teeth........, skin......... Abnormal lack of sweating........, oddly-shaped nose.........

e. Metabolic disorder symptoms: edema (around eyes)........, large tongue........, cool dry skin........, hernias........, muscle weakness

........, progressive ataxia.........

f. Other somatic disorder symptoms: low-set ears........, mental retardation........, facial capillary hemangioma........, polydactyly........, sloping forehead........, posterior prominence of heels........, low birth weight........, failure to thrive.........

10. Any of the following physical conditions which may be noted on chart but not obvious on simple inspection of infant:

a. Renal disorders: microscopic hematuria........, microscopic albuminuria........, ichthyosis ...., hyperprolinemia........, prolinuria........, hydroxyprolinuria........, glycinuria........, renal anomalies........, superimposed pyelonephritis ...., hematuria.........

b. Endocrine disorders: nonendemic goiter........, associated hypothyroidism........, diabetes mellitus........, optic atrophy.........

c. Heart disease symptoms: EKG abnormalities ...., congenital pulmonary stenosis........, hypertelorism.........

d. Degenerative disorders of nervous system: loss of reflexes........, nystagmus........, optic atrophy........, myoclonic seizures........, photomyoclonus........, cerebral dysfunction........,

e. Brain syndrome symptoms: spasticity........, seizures........, tremor........, homocystinemia ....

f. Other neurologic disorders: severe infantile muscular dystrophy........, difficulty eating ...., facial weakness........, hypoactive tendon reflexes.........

g. Unclassified: acute osteomyelitis........, recurrent pneumonia........, pulmonary disease ...., intestinal atresia........, uveitis........, parotitis........, dermatitis.........

[72]